Integrated Palliative Care of Respiratory Disease

Stephen J. Bourke • E. Timothy Peel
Editors

Integrated Palliative Care of Respiratory Disease

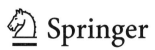 Springer

Editors
Stephen J. Bourke, M.D., FRCP, FRCPI, DCH
Department of Respiratory Medicine
Royal Victoria Infirmary
Newcastle upon Tyne
UK

E. Timothy Peel, M.B.B.S., B.Sc., FRCP
Department of Palliative Medicine
North Tyneside General Hospital
Rake Lane
North Shields
UK

Marie Curie Hospice
Newcastle upon Tyne
UK

ISBN 978-1-4471-2229-6   ISBN 978-1-4471-2230-2   (eBook)
DOI 10.1007/978-1-4471-2230-2
Springer London Heidelberg New York Dordrecht

Library of Congress Control Number: 2012950457

Printed on acid-free paper

Springer is part of Springer Science+Business Media (www.springer.com)

Preface

Palliative care of respiratory disease is often complex because of the high level of symptoms experienced by these patients and the variable and sometimes unpredictable trajectories of these diseases. Sudden death is a feature of catastrophic illnesses such as severe pneumonia or acute lung injury. The end of life phase may be short and is likely to be in the setting of an intensive care unit. A transplant trajectory is a particular feature for some lung diseases such as cystic fibrosis or idiopathic pulmonary fibrosis. The patient is seriously ill, has distressing symptoms, and may die but is hoping for a rescue lung transplant which can transform the trajectory of the disease. More commonly patients are living their lives with chronic progressive lung diseases such as chronic obstructive pulmonary disease, fibrotic lung disease, neuromuscular disease, or cystic fibrosis. They show considerable resilience and fortitude in coping with the disability and distress of a life-limiting condition. These diseases tend to progress, but often over a period of many years, and are characterized by acute exacerbations. Often treatment will reverse the exacerbation and restore health but an acute exacerbation may be the start of the dying phase of the disease, and it is important to recognize when this is happening. Admission to hospital may be the best way of bringing comfort and control to a patient experiencing severe distress because of an acute exacerbation or a complication such as pneumothorax, infection, or hemoptysis. Urgent assessment is required before deciding with the patient and family on the best course of action. It is clear that a traditional model of palliative care, based on a cancer trajectory which sometimes artificially divides care into a disease-modifying phase and a palliative phase, is often not appropriate for patients with chronic progressive lung disease. Care must be organized in such a way that disease-modifying treatments, supportive care, emergency care, palliative care, and end of life care all run in parallel. Flexibility is required to meet the needs of patients, and good quality care must be achieved in a variety of settings including the patient's home, care homes, clinics, emergency departments, medical wards, and ICUs.

Palliative care principles apply at all stages of serious disease and a major success has been the dissemination of the knowledge, skills, and ethos of palliative care to clinical teams in all areas of medical practice. Many patients with lung disease are cared for by a multidisciplinary team which strives to provide holistic care. It is often most appropriate to integrate palliative care into the multidisciplinary team with specialist palliative care clinicians working alongside the respiratory team. This encourages a focus on symptom management, supportive care, and quality of life at an earlier stage in the disease process, and can facilitate discussions about advanced care planning and end of life issues. As patients enter advanced stage disease, specialist palliative care skills may be needed in relieving complex symptoms and in ensuring optimal end of life care. Palliative care teams may be able to facilitate a patient's wish to be at home when dying or to give access to hospice care if appropriate. This model of integrated care provides continuity of care and makes it easier to manage any acute crisis which may occur in advanced lung disease.

This book brings together the knowledge and skills of specialists in both Respiratory Medicine and Palliative Medicine in an integrated approach to the care of patients with severe lung disease. We have much to learn from each other, and from our patients, who have much to gain from integrated collaborative models of palliative care.

Stephen J. Bourke, E. Timothy Peel

Contents

Contributors

Stephen C. Bourke, M.B. BCh, Ph.D., FRCP Department of Respiratory Medicine, North Tyneside General Hospital, North Shields, Tyne and Wear, UK

Stephen J. Bourke, M.D., FRCP, FRCPI, DCH Department of Respiratory Medicine, Royal Victoria Infirmary, Newcastle upon Tyne, UK

Graham P. Burns, B.Sc., M.B.B.S., FRCP, DipMedSci., Ph.D.
Department of Respiratory Medicine, Royal Victoria Infirmary,
Newcastle upon Tyne, UK

Ian A. Forrest, B.Sc., M.B. ChB, Ph.D. FRCP Department of Respiratory Medicine, Royal Victoria Infirmary, Newcastle upon Tyne, UK

Alistair D. Gascoigne, M.B.B.S., FRCP, B.Sc. Department of Critical Care Medicine, Royal Victoria Infirmary, Newcastle upon Tyne, UK

Eleanor Grogan, B.Sc., M.B.B.S., M.A., FRCP Department of Palliative Medicine, Wansbeck General Hospital, Northumberland, UK

Bernard Higgins, MB ChB (Hons), M.D., FRCP Department of Respiratory Medicine, Freeman Hospital, Newcastle upon Tyne, UK

Catherine O'Neill, M.B.B.S., MRCP Department of Palliative Medicine, Wansbeck General Hospital, Northumberland, UK

St Oswald's Hospice, Newcastle upon Tyne, UK

Paul Paes, M.B.B.S., M.Sc., MMedEd, FRCP Department of Palliative Care, Northumbria Healthcare NHS Foundation Trust, Newcastle University, North Shields, Tyne and Wear, UK

North Tyneside General Hospital, North Shields, Tyne and Wear, UK

E. Timothy Peel, M.B.B.S., B.Sc., FRCP Department of Palliative Medicine, North Tyneside General Hospital, North Shields, Tyne and Wear, UK

Marie Curie Hospice, Newcastle upon Tyne, UK

Rachel Quibell, M.B.B.S., FRCP Department of Palliative Medicine,
Royal Victoria Infirmary, Newcastle upon Tyne, UK

Chris Stenton, FRCP, FFOM Department of Respiratory Medicine,
Royal Victoria Infirmary, Newcastle upon Tyne, UK

Part I
Palliative Care Principles

Chapter 1
Palliative Care of Respiratory Disease

Stephen J. Bourke and E. Timothy Peel

Abstract Respiratory disease is a major cause of suffering and death. There is a broad range of disease from acute illnesses such as pneumonia and acute lung injury to chronic progressive diseases such as chronic obstructive lung disease, cystic fibrosis, and neuromuscular disease. The different trajectories of lung disease are outlined including sudden death from catastrophic illness, the cancer trajectory in patients with lung cancer, the chronic disease trajectory for patients with progressive lung diseases, and the transplant trajectory for patients with diseases such as cystic fibrosis or idiopathic pulmonary fibrosis. Palliative and supportive care run in parallel with disease-modifying therapies throughout the course of life-threatening respiratory disease. A multidisciplinary integrated approach is needed in treating these patients and good quality palliative care must be achieved in a variety of settings including the patient's home, care homes, clinics, emergency departments, wards, and intensive care units.

Keywords Palliative care respiratory disease • Disease trajectories • Lung transplantation • Hospice • Palliative medicine • Multidisciplinary

S.J. Bourke, M.D., FRCP, FRCPI, DCH (✉)
Department of Respiratory Medicine, Royal Victoria Infirmary,
Queen Victoria Road, Newcastle upon Tyne NE1 4LP, UK
e-mail: stephen.bourke@nuth.nhs.uk

E.T. Peel, M.B.B.S., B.Sc., FRCP
Department of Palliative Medicine, North Tyneside General Hospital,
Rake Lane, North Shields, Tyne and Wear NE29 8NH, UK

Marie Curie Hospice,
Newcastle upon Tyne, UK

S.J. Bourke, E.T. Peel (eds.), *Integrated Palliative Care of Respiratory Disease*,
DOI 10.1007/978-1-4471-2230-2_1, © Springer-Verlag London 2013

3

One of the major successes of modern Medicine has been the development of palliative medicine as a specialty in its own right and the dissemination of the knowledge, skills, and ethos of palliative care to clinical teams in all areas of medical practice [1]. This is particularly the case in respiratory medicine where considerable progress has been made in supporting patients living their lives with chronic lung disease, in relieving symptoms at all stages of a disease process and in providing end of life care to patients facing death [2].

The modern era of palliative medicine started in the second half of the twentieth century with an initial focus on the degree of distress suffered by patients dying of cancer. Key pioneers were Dame Cicely Saunders who founded St Christopher's Hospice, London, in 1967, and Elisabeth Kübler-Ross, who conducted interviews with patients who were dying, leading to her seminal publication *On Death and Dying* in 1970 [1, 3, 4]. These pioneers of palliative care built on the earlier successes of previous hospices such as Our Lady's Hospice in Dublin, which was established in 1879, and St. Joseph's Hospice in East London, established in 1902. Care of patients in their own homes was a feature of the hospice movement from the start with a philosophy that hospice care was a concept rather than merely a place of care. Early developments were the extension of home-care and the establishment of hospital-care teams visiting patients across all specialties to bring the skills of palliative care to seriously ill hospitalized patients. Palliative Medicine gained formal recognition as a specialty in 1987 in the United Kingdom (UK), Australia, and New Zealand, and subsequently in the United States of America (USA) in 2007. This led to the establishment of formal training programmes, the expansion of clinical services, and the development of research in all areas of palliative care.

Initially the focus was on patients dying of cancer but it rapidly became clear that those dying from other chronic diseases also had considerable palliative care needs [5–8]. Furthermore, there was an important role in the relief of symptoms and the provision of support at all stages of serious illness, not merely in those approaching death. The World Health Organization defined palliative care as an approach that improves the quality of life of patients and their families facing the problems associated with life-threatening illness [9]. Key elements of palliative care include the relief of symptoms and distress, a team approach in addressing the needs of patients and their families, the enhancement of life, the mitigation of suffering, and the recognition of dying as a normal process bringing life to a natural end. Death should not necessarily be regarded as a "failure of Medicine" but that "a good natural death" should be seen as a key goal of medical care.

There have been many further developments in palliative medicine over the years but the major current focus is on extending the ethos of palliative care to all clinical teams in all areas of medical practice with palliative care running in parallel with disease-modifying therapies throughout the course of a disease. In 2008, the American Thoracic Society endorsed the concept that palliative care should be available to patients at all stages of illness and that clinicians who care for patients with chronic or advanced respiratory disease should have training and competencies in palliative care and access to consultations with palliative care specialists and services [10]. In the UK, the Department of Health published its strategy for dealing with end of life care in 2008 and the National Institute for Health and Clinical Excellence published its quality standards for end of life care in 2011 [11, 12]. The emphasis of these initiatives is on predicting the prognosis of a disease, recognizing that the patient is entering the end of life phase (the last 6–12 months) and catering for their particular needs at this time.

Extent of Respiratory Disease

Respiratory disease is a major cause of suffering and death throughout the world, accounting for about four million deaths each year. For some diseases, the prevalence and mortality are rising [13]. This is particularly the case for chronic obstructive pulmonary disease (COPD). In the USA, for example, the death rate from COPD doubled over a 40 year period [14]. In Europe, there are about 390,000 new cases of lung cancer each year and it is the major cause of cancer death [13]. In the UK, about 20 % of all deaths are due to lung disease. There are about 34,000 deaths each year from pneumonia, 33,000 deaths from lung cancer, 30,000 deaths from COPD, and 2,500 deaths from occupational lung diseases such as mesothelioma and pneumoconiosis [15].

There is a broad range of respiratory disease from acute illnesses such as pneumonia, asthma, and acute lung injury to chronic progressive diseases such as COPD, fibrotic lung disease, cystic fibrosis, and neuromuscular disease. About 10 % of all patients in hospital suffer from a respiratory illness. About 6 % of the UK population are living their lives with a long-term respiratory disease, rising to about 10 % of those over the age of 65 years [15].

Symptoms of Respiratory Disease

Patients with lung disease often have a high level of severe symptoms such as breathlessness, cough, respiratory secretions, and pain [2, 6, 10]. For many patients with chronic lung disease, breathlessness is a dominant symptom which is difficult to relieve. Optimal disease-modifying measures, pulmonary rehabilitation, and appropriate use of oxygen may all improve breathlessness but reduced exercise capacity with associated breathlessness is often an inherent feature of lung diseases such as idiopathic pulmonary fibrosis and COPD. Opiate and benzodiazepine medications may help reduce the sensation of breathlessness but in many patients it is not possible to fully relieve this symptom, and patients are likely to need additional measures to support them in coping with activities of daily living. They have substantial disability which often leads to a vicious cycle of breathlessness, reduced physical activities and deconditioning of muscles with secondary problems of social isolation, loss of autonomy, depression, and anxiety. They often have a complex range of emotional responses to their illness such as frustration, anxiety, panic, and fear of the future. The emotional and psychological impact of chronic lung disease can be as severe as the physical symptoms. Many patients with lung disease have to cope with complex and intrusive treatments which may include multiple drug treatments, nebulized medications, physiotherapy, oxygen therapy, and in some cases non-invasive ventilation and nutritional support. Patients are often living their lives in the knowledge of having a chronic life-limiting disease. As a disease progresses, it is often necessary to intensify treatments but an ever-increasing treatment burden can further impair quality of life. Skills from several disciplines are needed in treating these patients and a multidisciplinary integrated approach is essential. Typically this currently involves doctors, specialist nurses, physiotherapists, and social workers and may increasingly involve palliative care clinicians, particularly as the focus changes in the course of the disease from chronic disease management to end of life care. End of life care includes the last phase of an illness, often extending over the last 6–12 months of life, rather than being confined to the terminal hours or days. In addition to expert treatment directed against the disease process, patients often benefit from supportive measures to enable them to live in their own home, pulmonary rehabilitation to improve the quality of life and psychological therapies, such as cognitive behavioral therapy to help them cope with and adjust to living with a chronic progressive lung disease. Many patients with chronic lung disease are elderly and suffer from general frailty and additional comorbid conditions, such that several disease processes may be present in an individual patient [16].

Respiratory Disease Trajectories (Fig. 1.1)

Predicting the prognosis of lung disease is often difficult and it is sometimes necessary for the patient and the clinical team to accept uncertainty. The rate at which a disease progresses – the disease trajectory – is often highly variable in chronic lung disease and patients follow their own unique clinical course [17–19]. Sudden death is a feature of catastrophic illnesses such as severe pneumonia or acute lung injury. The end of life phase may be short, often over a few hours, and is likely to be in the setting of an intensive care unit (ICU). In contrast, patients with lung cancer often follow the "cancer trajectory" where there is an initial phase of disease-modifying treatments such as chemotherapy and radiotherapy, followed by a phase of progression of the cancer and declining health, evolving into a clearer palliative phase culminating in end of life care which may be in a hospice or in the patient's home, for example. However, this traditional model of palliative care often does not fit well with chronic lung disease, where the clinical course is more variable. Patients live their lives with the disability and distress of a chronic illness which cannot be cured and in the knowledge that this is a life-limiting condition. However, a patient's life span after diagnosis can be decades. Patients with diseases such as COPD, cystic fibrosis, or neuromuscular disease show considerable resilience and fortitude under these circumstances. In most cases, palliative care runs in parallel with disease-modifying treatments, supportive care and measures aimed at improving quality of

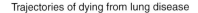

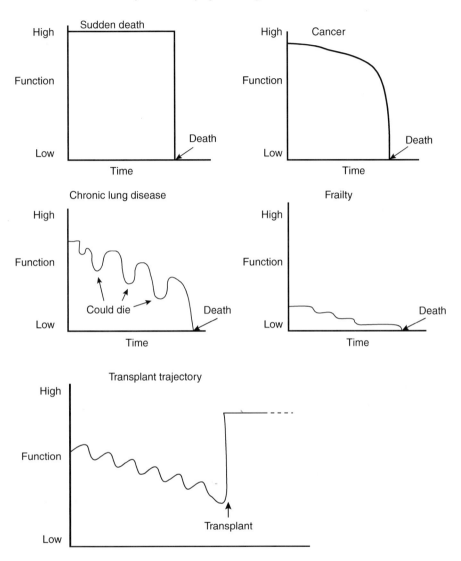

Fig. 1.1 Trajectories of dying from lung disease. The rate at which lung diseases progress is highly variable. Sudden death is a feature of catastrophic illnesses such as severe pneumonia. Lung cancer often follows a typical cancer trajectory. Chronic lung diseases such as COPD are characterized by gradual progression with intermittent exacerbations. Many patients with COPD are elderly with progressive frailty. A transplant trajectory is a particular feature of some lung diseases such as cystic fibrosis

life. Many chronic lung diseases are characterized by acute exacerbations that can be reversed by acute treatments, which often involve admission to hospital. It is important to appreciate that acute exacerbations usually cause severe symptoms such as breathlessness, cough, pain, and distress which require emergency treatment. Such treatments not only reverse the underlying disease process but are the most effective way of relieving symptoms. Thus, a course of intravenous antibiotics, with oxygen and sputum clearance physiotherapy, is the most effective way of relieving symptoms in a patient with an exacerbation of cystic fibrosis lung disease. Patients may suffer acute complications in the course of chronic lung disease, such as pneumothorax, pneumonia, or major hemoptysis, which cause an acute crisis with severe distress, that can be relieved by prompt diagnosis and expert interventions. Such complications are more likely to occur in advanced-stage disease, and can be very difficult to manage well if an artificial model is followed, whereby palliative care is separated from active disease-modifying care. Such models of care provision are usually inappropriate for patients with progressive lung disease. It is usually better to organize care in such a way that disease-modifying treatments, emergency interventions for any acute crisis, and palliative and supportive measures run in parallel.

Patients with COPD typically have a trajectory of gradual decline punctuated by episodes of acute deterioration and recovery with treatment. The end of life phase is not clearly defined. The patient recovers from all acute exacerbations except the final one, and death can then be somewhat unexpected. This is sometimes referred to as "acute crisis/recovery trajectory." Many patients with chronic lung disease are elderly and frail with comorbid conditions [16]. They may suffer dwindling health with increasing difficulties in coping at home even with intensive support, such that they may decide to live in a care home, which provides a high level of nursing and supportive care. Such patients may be following a chronic lung disease trajectory, but death may occur from other causes such as a myocardial infarction or stroke [6].

A "transplant trajectory" is a particular feature for some lung diseases such as cystic fibrosis, idiopathic pulmonary fibrosis, primary pulmonary hypertension, or emphysema due to alpha-one-antitrypsin deficiency, for example. The patient is seriously ill, has a high level of symptoms, and may die but is hoping for a rescue lung transplant which can transform the trajectory of the disease dramatically.

Other trajectories may apply to specific aspects of a disease. For example, emotional distress tends to peak at the time of diagnosis of a serious disease, such as lung cancer, at times of deterioration or relapse, and as death approaches. At the time of diagnosis the patient has to cope with the communication of bad news and adjust to living with a serious life-limiting disease. There are elements of grief and loss at this time.

There are substantial limitations to predicting the disease trajectory in patients with lung disease but there may be some advantage in predicting that a patient is likely to die within "months rather than years" or within 6 months, as this may avoid "prognostic paralysis" and may allow access to some additional support services. In some healthcare systems, particular services or financial support are made available to patients who are unlikely to survive more than 6 months. For some diseases, such as lung cancer or progressive idiopathic pulmonary fibrosis, the disease trajectory is generally more predictable, and this facilitates discussion of prognosis and end of life planning. For other patients, such as those with COPD or cystic fibrosis, it is necessary to acknowledge uncertainty. The prognosis and future plans can be discussed in terms of what is likely to happen over a period of time, but precise planning is often unhelpful and plans need to be adaptable to deal with events.

Integrating Palliative Care into Respiratory Care

Palliative care of respiratory disease is highly complex and no one model of care will suit all patients. Different countries organize their palliative care services in different ways but good quality care must be achieved in a variety of settings including the patient's home, care homes, clinics, emergency departments, specialist respiratory wards, and ICUs. Delivery of care will depend on the patient's needs, the skills of the clinical team, and the availability of specialist palliative services. It is now widely recognized that palliative care principles apply at all stages of disease and that all doctors and clinical teams should be able to recognize the patient's needs and to deliver general palliative care, including elements of symptom control, support, communication, and discussion of future care planning. Specialists in palliative medicine have a crucial role in providing education and support to these clinical teams, with collaborative working across traditional boundaries.

There are substantial differences in the use of specialist palliative care services between patients with cancer and patients with other chronic lung diseases [6–8]. Surveys have shown that only a minority of patients dying with chronic lung disease have had input from specialist palliative care services [20]. This could be due to many factors including the clinical course followed by the disease, a failure to refer patients to palliative services, a reluctance of palliative services to be involved with these patients, or a reluctance of the patients to consider palliative care. These are complex issues and the best way of providing palliative care to these patients has not yet been established. Many of these patients have longstanding relationships with a multidisciplinary respiratory team which endeavors to provide holistic care. Patients often value this continuity of care and it is not clear that their needs are best met by a transfer of care from respiratory services to palliative services, especially when disease-modifying therapies, emergency treatments, and palliative care need to run in parallel. This is particularly the case in specialist areas such as cystic fibrosis, fibrotic lung disease, and neuromuscular disease for example. It is often more appropriate to integrate palliative care and specialist respiratory care, with members of the palliative care team working within the respiratory multidisciplinary team. As such patients enter advanced stage disease, particular palliative care skills may be needed in relieving complex symptoms and in addressing end of life issues. Specialist palliative care services may be able to facilitate a patient's wish to be at home when dying or to give access to hospice care if appropriate. Community-based hospice teams are increasingly able to provide high-intensity palliative care in the patient's home. In this integrated model of collaborative working between respiratory and palliative care teams, it is easier to manage any acute crises or complications which may arise in advanced lung disease. Integrated palliative care also encourages a focus on symptom management, support, communication, and quality of life issues at an earlier stage in the disease process. Respiratory teams may be highly focused on specific disease-modifying treatments and parameters such as lung function, and traditionally have been less focused on balancing the burden of treatment against the burden of disease, although increasingly quality of life is being assessed as a key outcome measure of any treatment. Respiratory teams may be reluctant to discuss prognosis and future planning in detail. Some studies suggest that patients want to make plans for their future care and would like their clinical teams to start such discussions. Palliative care clinicians can facilitate such discussions. Sometimes a question such as "what worries you most about the future?" can be a useful way of approaching the subject. There may be key events which should trigger these discussions such as an admission to hospital with an exacerbation of COPD, an episode of respiratory failure requiring non-invasive ventilation, or a deterioration in lung function in a progressive respiratory disease. Some patients have particular fears which can be addressed and alleviated. For example, patients who have problems with respiratory secretions may fear that they will choke to death and breathless patients may fear that death will be painful with them struggling to breathe [21]. They can be reassured that such symptoms can be controlled. Palliative care clinicians working within respiratory teams can help to identify patients with additional needs for specialist palliative care input and services.

It is particularly important that palliative care has a high profile in certain areas such as ICU, emergency departments, and acute medicine wards. Because acute exacerbations and complications often occur in advanced lung disease, these patients require access to emergency services. Prompt assessment is required to identify the problem and urgent specific treatment is needed to deal with complications such as infection, hemoptysis, and pneumothorax. In many cases, accurate diagnosis and specific treatment will relieve symptoms and lead to recovery from the acute crisis. However, an acute crisis may be the start of the dying process for these patients. If disease-modifying treatments are failing and the patient is progressively deteriorating, it is important to recognize when the patient is dying and when escalation of treatments such as invasive ventilation may be futile and not in the patient's best interests. It is crucial that patients, their relatives, and the general public have confidence in the ability of emergency services to provide urgent palliation and that the general public do not develop erroneous concepts of death in hospital being an undignified, painful struggle with high-technology intrusive treatments being applied inappropriately. One of the major successes in recent times has been the restoration of the caring role of clinical teams in managing a dying patient, with the progress in palliative care as a specialty. There is sometimes an inappropriate concept that patients in the palliative stages of a disease should not be admitted to an acute hospital. Acute palliative care is a key component of emergency medicine and these patients often need emergency assessment and management during an acute crisis and hospital is often the best place to achieve this, and should not be denied to the patient. This may be the best way of bringing comfort and control to a patient and family in severe distress because of an acute crisis in the course of a progressive lung disease.

Particular consideration is needed in deciding how to organize urgent care for individual patients when a crisis occurs in their advanced stage disease. It is helpful if discussions have taken place in advance about potential options and "ceilings of care," whereby some complications are treatable offering the possibility of recovery but that other treatments may not be feasible or may be futile. An acute crisis in the course of chronic lung disease often causes acute severe breathlessness, which is very distressing for patients and their families. Ideally admission to hospital should be directly to the clinical team which knows them well. Thus a patient with cystic fibrosis or neuromuscular disease, for example, develops a crisis and contacts their specialist team who arranges urgent assessment, diagnoses the problem, and decides with the patient on the best course of action. This can result in rapid control of a situation in which the patient and family are very distressed. It is more difficult to organize such a level of care for diseases such as COPD where there are large numbers of patients. It is helpful if there is clear detailed documentation of the patient's baseline status so that decisions can be made rapidly as to what is the most appropriate course of action to be taken in the context of the current crisis. It is important that there has been good communication and sharing of information with the patient, the family, and all involved in the patient's care. Any advanced care directives must be clearly documented. There will still often be a need for emergency assessment of the current problem with further discussion with the patient and family about the treatment options, leading to a decision about the best course of action. When these patients have failed to respond to treatment and are entering the dying phase, it is important to make the specific diagnosis that the patient is now dying, so that care can be focused on management of the dying patient and their family, often using a care pathway such as the Liverpool care pathway [22]. It is crucial that this is a positive diagnosis leading to urgent end of life management, rather than a negative attitude of "there is nothing more we can do." There may be only a short time in which there is the opportunity to achieve the key goal of "a good death" for the patient without the opportunity to subsequently correct any deficiencies in care [23, 24]. These patients often have substantial symptoms such as breathlessness, which need urgent relief. Delay in diagnosing the dying phase can result in inadequate symptom control. In most hospitals, palliative care teams are available to support the clinical team in managing such patients and their families. Paradoxically these patients have often had a prolonged palliative phase to their disease during which they have been living their lives with substantial disability, but the timing of terminal stage disease is unpredictable and the terminal phase is often short. This pattern is often discussed with the patients in terms of "keeping you as well as possible for as long as possible, and comfortable when the time comes." Providing palliative care for this disease trajectory is particularly important for many chronic lung diseases.

Patients with lung cancer often follow a traditional palliative care trajectory, and it may be more appropriate to transfer their care from an oncology team to a palliative care team as the disease progresses and as death approaches. Nevertheless in the UK and many other countries, these patients often have continuity of care provided by a Respiratory Physician or by their primary care general practitioner. Palliative care is an integral part of the general care of patients at all stages of respiratory disease and they should have access to specialist palliative care services according to their needs and wishes. Considerable flexibility is need in providing palliative care to these patients.

Terminology and Definitions

There are some terms and phrases which are commonly used to describe the interventions and approaches to the care of patients with progressive disease:

Palliative care: It is an approach that focuses on the total care of the patient and family who are facing life-threatening illness [9]. It embraces symptom control, psychological, social, and spiritual support and aims to optimize quality of life in those with an incurable illness. This type of care should be offered by all healthcare professionals.

Specialist palliative care: It is care provided by clinicians who have specialist training and skills in palliative medicine, working within specialist multidisciplinary teams.

Supportive care: It is a broader concept which includes the provision of support and palliation to patients at an earlier stage of their illness when outcomes, such as cure, are still possible.

Disease-modifying treatment: It refers to treatments of the underlying condition that may halt or slow the disease process. In terms of an ultimately fatal disease such as mesothelioma, chemotherapy might be expected to prolong survival as well as improving symptoms. Disease modification may be achieved with drugs, lifestyle changes, such as smoking-cessation in COPD, and non-drug interventions such as radiotherapy in lung cancer.

Active treatment: It includes both disease-modifying treatments and a range of possible interventions for potential complications which may arise. Examples might include antibiotics for intercurrent infections or mucolytics and physiotherapy for sputum clearance. Active treatment and palliative care are not mutually exclusive.

Ceilings of care: It is a phrase used to describe what interventions might be appropriate and desirable depending on the circumstances which might arise when an outcome of an illness is unpredictable. This is a management plan by the clinical team, taking into account the wishes of the patient and family. Sometimes called treatment escalation plans, examples of ceiling of care options include, at one end of the spectrum whether to use antibiotics for an infection, and at the other whether a patient should be transferred to the ICU for ventilation for respiratory failure. Examples of ceilings of care include the following:

- Lung transplantation
- Cardiopulmonary resuscitation and invasive ventilation
- Non-invasive ventilation

- Clinically assisted nutrition
- Clinically assisted hydration
- Surgery if otherwise indicated, such as for an acute abdominal condition
- Intravenous antibiotics
- Oral antibiotics
- Disease-modifying drugs
- Symptom-controlling measures only

In the context of advanced respiratory disease, it is important to stress that however actively the disease is to be managed, palliative treatments should still be offered if necessary. Similarly palliative care does not imply withdrawal of disease-modifying treatment. Guidance has been published by the General Medical Council in the UK on decision making at the end of life [25]. Patients may refuse a proposed treatment if they have capacity to make the decision or if they have made an advanced directive to refuse treatment. If a patient lacks capacity and has already appointed a legal proxy, then that person can refuse the proposed treatment on behalf of the patient. If the patient requests a treatment which the doctor, after due consideration, does not think is clinically appropriate, the doctor is not beholden to provide that treatment but is advised to seek consensus, to discuss the reasons for the decision and to offer a second opinion.

Prescribing in Palliative Care

Licensed, Unlicensed, and Off-label Drugs

In the UK, drugs can be licensed either through the European Medicines Agency (EMA) or the Medicines and Healthcare Products Regulatory Agency (MRHA). Drugs are licensed for a specific indication and administration route (e.g., oral or subcutaneous injection). Most drugs are therefore prescribed according to license (indication and route), for example morphine sulphate modified release tablets orally for pain. There are also some unlicensed preparations available, such as cyclizine suppositories for nausea and vomiting. Finally, and most commonly seen in palliative medicine practice, is the use of a licensed drug for an indication outside the license, or given by an unlicensed route. This is commonly referred to as off-label or off-license prescribing. Appendix B lists some unlicensed drugs and off-license prescribing. The General Medical Council gives guidance on unlicensed and off-license prescribing [26]. Both are permissible if the prescriber is satisfied that the drug would serve the patient's needs better than licensed preparations, that there is sufficient evidence of efficacy and safety, and that the prescriber will oversee the patient's care and document the reasons for the prescription. This should also be discussed with the patient.

Opioid Prescribing Issues

Opioid dose conversions: It is often necessary to change one opioid drug to another, either because of adverse effects or lack of benefit. Recommended conversion ratios used in this book are based on recent European Association for Palliative Care guidelines, and are in line with other guidance [27, 28]. In two cases, these differ from the manufacturer's suggestions (morphine-oxycodone and morphine-fentanyl conversions). It is important to appreciate that there is significant individual variation in the pharmacokinetics of these drugs between patients such that conversion ratios are approximations and may not be equi-analgesic, and further titration may be necessary.

Rescue doses: When prescribing a regular modified release opioid, it is important also to prescribe rescue (as necessary) analgesia for any breakthrough pain. This is usually prescribed hourly in hospices or hospitals and 4 hourly in the community (where there may be less ability to monitor toxicity). This is calculated by determining the total 24 hourly modified release dose and multiplying it by 1/10–1/6 to obtain the rescue dose of immediate release medication. The range allows doses in "round numbers."

Dose escalation: When pain is uncontrolled and the opioids are being escalated day on day, it is usual to increase the regular daily dose by 1/3–1/2 each time. The range allows calculation of doses in whole numbers. When the regular drug is increased, the rescue dose must also be increased. This is discussed further in Chap. 5.

References

1. Saunders C. The evolution of palliative care. J R Soc Med. 2001;94:430–2.
2. Selecky PA, Eliasson H, Hall RI, Schneider F, Varkey B, McCaffree DR. Palliative and end-of-life care for patients with cardiopulmonary diseases. Chest. 2005;128:3599–610.
3. Clemens KE, Klaschnik E. The history of hospice. In: Walsh D, editor. Palliative medicine. Philadelphia: Saunders/Elsevier; 2009. p. 18–23.
4. Kübler-Ross E. On death and dying. London: Tavistock Publication Ltd.; 1970.
5. Murtagh FEM, Preston M, Higginson I. Patterns of dying: palliative care for non-malignant disease. Clin Med. 2004;4:39–44.
6. Halpin DM, Seamark DA, Seamark CJ. Palliative and end-of-life care for patients with respiratory disease. Eur Respir Mon. 2009;43:327–53.
7. Davies L. Integrated care of the patient dying of nonmalignant respiratory disease. Breathe. 2008;5:155–61.
8. Gore JM, Brophy CJ, Greenstone MA. How well do we care for patients with end stage chronic obstructive pulmonary disease? A comparison of palliative care and quality of life in COPD and lung cancer. Thorax. 2000;55:1000–6.
9. World Health Organization definition of palliative care. WHO. http://www.who.int/cancer/palliative/definition/en/. Accessed 1 Apr 2012.
10. Lanken PN, Terry PB, DeLisser HM, et al. An official American Thoracic Society clinical policy statement: palliative care for patients with respiratory diseases and critical illnesses. Am J Respir Crit Care Med. 2008;177:912–27.
11. Richards M. End of life care strategy. London: Department of Health; 2008. www.dh.gov.uk/en/Healthcare/IntegratedCare/Endoflifecare/index.htm. Accessed 1 Apr 2012.

12. National Institute for Health and Clinical Excellence. End of life care for adults quality standards. NICE; 2011. http://www.nice.org.uk/guidance/qualitystandards/endoflifecare/. Accessed 1 Apr 2012.
13. Decramer M, Sibille Y, Nicod LP, et al. European Respiratory Roadmap 2011. European Respiratory Society 2011. http://www.ersroadmap.org/index. Accessed 1 Apr 2012.
14. Jemal A, Ward E, Hao Y, Thun M. Trends in the leading causes of death in the United States, 1970-2002. JAMA. 2005;294:1255–9.
15. British Thoracic Society. The burden of lung disease. London: British Thoracic Society; 2006. www.brit-thoracic.org.uk/library-guidelines/bts-publications/burden-of-lung-disease-reports. aspx#Burden1. Accessed 1 Apr 2012.
16. Clegg A, Young J. The frailty syndrome. Clin Med. 2011;11:72–5.
17. Murray SA, Kendall M, Boyd K, Dheikh A. Illness trajectories and palliative care. BMJ. 2005;330:1007–11.
18. Currow DC, Snith J, Davidson PM, Newton PJ, Agar MR, Abernethy AP. Do the trajectories of dyspnea differ in prevalence and intensity by diagnosis at the end of life? A consecutive cohort study. J Pain Symptom Manage. 2010;39:680–90.
19. Lunney JR, Lynn J, Foley DJ, Lipson S, Guralnik JM. Patterns of functional decline at the end of life. JAMA. 2003;289:2387–92.
20. Partridge MR, Khatri A, Sutton L, Welham S, Ahmedzai SH. Palliative care services for those with chronic lung disease. Chron Respir Dis. 2009;6:13–7.
21. Bourke SJ, Doe SJ, Gascoigne AD, et al. An integrated model of provision of palliative care to patients with cystic fibrosis. Palliat Med. 2009;23:512–7.
22. Ellershaw J, Foster A, Murphy D, Shea T, Overill S. Developing an integrated care pathway for the dying patient. Eur J Palliat Care. 1997;4:203–7.
23. Gibbins J, McCoubrie R, Alexander N, Kinzel C, Forbes K. Diagnosing dying in the acute hospital setting – are we too late? Clin Med. 2009;9:116–9.
24. Weissman DE, Meier DE. Identifying patients in need of a palliative care assessment in the hospital setting. J Palliat Med. 2011;14:17–22.
25. General Medical Council. Treatment and care towards the end of life: good practice in decision making. London: GMC; 2010. http://www.gmc-uk.org/End_of_life.pdf_32486688.pdf. Accessed 1 Apr 2012.
26. General Medical Council. Good practice in prescribing medicine – guidance for doctors. 2008. http://www.gmc-uk.org/guidance/ethical_guidance/prescriptions. Accessed 1 Apr 2012.
27. Caraceni A, Hanks G, Kassa S, et al. Use of opioid analgesics in the treatment of cancer pain: evidence-based recommendations from EAPC. Lancet Oncol. 2012;13:58–68.
28. Opioid dose conversion ratios. 2012. http://www.palliativedrugs.com. Accessed 1 Apr 2012.

Part II
Respiratory Symptoms

Chapter 2
Breathlessness

E. Timothy Peel and Graham P. Burns

Abstract Breathlessness is a complex symptom, incorporating physical and emotional components. After considering the control of respiration, the causes of breathlessness and mechanisms in chronic lung disease are described. The assessment of the breathlessness patient can include symptom scoring, measures of the impact on life, descriptors of the sensation and functional measures. Management is initially by disease modification of the underlying process, but alongside this, pharmacological and non-pharmacological interventions may be included. The principal drugs employed are opioids and benzodiazepines. There are a variety of non-drug interventions that are used for dyspnea in lung disease, some including an exercise component, some not. Oxygen also has a role in the hypoxemic patient. The presence of breathlessness can also have prognostic significance in advanced lung disease.

Keywords Breathlessness • Dyspnea • Assessment • Disease modification • Drug management • Non-pharmacological management

E.T. Peel, M.B.B.S., B.Sc., FRCP(✉)
Department of Palliative Medicine, North Tyneside General Hospital,
Rake Lane, North Shields, Tyne and Wear NE29 8NH, UK

Marie Curie Hospice,
Newcastle upon Tyne, UK
e-mail: tim.peel@northumbria-healthcare.nhs.uk

G.P. Burns, B.Sc., M.B.B.S., FRCP, DipMedSci., Ph.D.
Department of Respiratory Medicine, Royal Victoria Infirmary,
Queen Victoria Road, Newcastle upon Tyne NE1 4LP, UK

S.J. Bourke, E.T. Peel (eds.), *Integrated Palliative Care of Respiratory Disease*,
DOI 10.1007/978-1-4471-2230-2_2, © Springer-Verlag London 2013

Definition

Breathlessness, also known as dyspnea, is a symptom unique to the patient. Definitions stress the combination of unpleasant physical sensations with adverse emotions, such as anxiety, panic, or low mood [1]. The sensation of dyspnea arises as a result of complex synthesis of afferent signals to the brain, influenced by psychological and emotional factors and interpreted subconsciously based on a bench marking of past experience. Because of the close association between physical and emotional inputs, it is often difficult to separate cause and effect in the anxious breathless patient.

Breathlessness is not the same as:

Tachypnea. An increased rate of breathing.

Hyperventilation. "Over ventilation" of (the alveoli) beyond the level needed to maintain a normal pCO_2. Many doctors tend to use the term loosely to mean "anxiety-driven hyperventilation." It should be noted that anxiety is far from the only cause of a diminished pCO_2. Care is needed so that causes such as pulmonary embolism, acute severe asthma, and metabolic acidosis are not mistaken for "mere anxiety."

Control of Breathing

For most people, in health, breathing is an automatic function, controlled by the autonomic nervous system, and does not impact on consciousness. If we deliberately turn our attention to it, however, it can be readily perceived. The four respiratory centers are located in the brainstem (medulla and pons). They receive information from a number of central and peripheral receptors. Central chemoreceptors are located in the medulla and respond to changes in pCO_2 and therefore pH. Peripheral chemoreceptors are in the carotid and aortic bodies and respond to changes in pO_2. There are also stretch receptors in the chest wall muscles, mechanoreceptors in the airways and lung parenchyma, and also temperature receptors in the airways. These all transmit afferent messages to the respiratory centers where ventilation is controlled. This dictates the necessary ventilatory rate and depth via the common efferent pathway.

When the respiratory motor center sends an efferent signal to the respiratory muscles, it sends a copy of the signal (corollary discharge) [2] to perceptual areas in higher centers. The brain thus knows "what has been asked" of the ventilatory system. This information is compared with information returning from the respiratory muscles and other afferent signals on what is being achieved in terms of ventilation. When these two match, no red flags are raised, breathing continues automatically, essentially unnoticed. When a mismatch occurs, when the return on effort is not what it should be the individual experiences an uncomfortable sense of inappropriate respiratory effort, more usually described as "breathlessness." Mismatch could be due to

Table 2.1 Breathlessness: causes

Respiratory		
Chronic	COPD/asthma	
	Sepsis	Bronchiectasis
		Cystic fibrosis
	Cancer	Lung cancer
		Mesothelioma
		Intrathoracic metastases
	Fibrosis	
	Respiratory muscle weakness due to cachexia	
	Neuromuscular	Motor neurone disease
		Muscular dystrophies
	Skeletal	Chest wall abnormalities
Acute	Pneumonia	
	Emphysema	
	Pneumothorax	
Pulmonary vascular	Pulmonary thromboembolism: acute and chronic (recurrent)	
	Pulmonary hypertension: primary and secondary	
Cardiac		
Chronic	Heart failure (right, left, or congestive)	
	Arrhythmias (particularly atrial fibrillation)	
Acute	Coronary events	
Psychological	Anxiety, depression, hyperventilation	
Anemia		
Cachexia		

a number of mechanisms impeding the ventilatory response to its neurological command: obstruction to airflow, increased load on respiratory muscles (including hyperinflation see below), or respiratory muscle weakness.

Descending pathways, either via the thalamus or directly to the respiratory muscles, are the means whereby we can, to some extent, voluntarily alter our pattern of breathing.

Most of the drugs that are used for purely symptomatic relief of dyspnea act at the higher centers.

Causes

There are many causes of breathlessness, both acute and chronic. Some of these are primarily due to underlying respiratory disease, whilst others are a manifestation of pulmonary vascular, cardiac, psychological, or other diseases. The causes are summarized in Table 2.1. The medical treatment of many of these underlying conditions (i.e., disease modification) is not within the scope of this chapter. When describing management options for dyspnea, it is assumed that all appropriate medical treatments for the underlying cause have been offered.

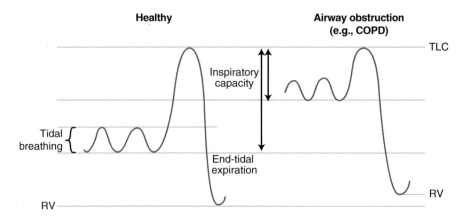

Fig. 2.1 Graph of lung volumes against time in a healthy subject and a patient with airway obstruction (e.g., COPD). In the context of COPD, tidal breathing occurs at a higher lung volume; this helps to support the airway open but has a number of other consequences (see text). Note the inspiratory capacity (the gap between the lung volume at the end of a tidal expiration and the total lung capacity) is reduced in airway obstruction. *TLC* total lung capacity, *RV* residual volume

Mechanisms of Dyspnea in Chronic Lung Disease

Hyperinflation

In diseases that cause airway obstruction, for example, asthma and chronic obstructive pulmonary disease (COPD), in an attempt to obviate the degree of airway narrowing, patients tend to breathe at a higher lung volume; closer to total lung capacity (TLC) than usual (Fig. 2.1). In this way lung tissue is stretched and the airways that are embedded within it experience a greater retractile force and are, to some extent, widened. In that sense the strategy works. This, of course, is not a deliberate or even conscious change; patients are unaware that they are breathing at a higher lung volume. There are a number of other consequences to this adaptation which can give rise to specific symptoms. As can be seen, breathing at a higher lung volume implies that the inspiratory capacity is diminished. Therefore, if a patient attempts to take a deep breath in, they will find they reach their limit (TLC) sooner than expected. Unaware that their inspiratory maneuver began at a high lung volume and unaware that they are already at TLC, this limitation to further inspiration will be perceived as an "inability to get a full breath in."

In healthy subjects at the end of a normal tidal expiration, the intrinsic tendency for the lungs to contract is just counterbalanced by the natural tendency for the chest wall to "spring outward." No muscular effort (no work) is required to hold this "neutral" position. Breathing close to this lung volume is therefore quite effort efficient, like gently stretching and releasing a spring that has no baseline tension. As lung volume increases, lung tissue is stretched, and like the spring it tends to resist further stretch. In fact, unlike the perfect spring of Hooke's law, the greater the stretch, the greater the force that is required to further expand the lung. When, as in airway obstruction, tidal breathing occurs at a higher lung volume, the muscular effort needed simply to move the chest wall (*the work of breathing*) is hugely increased. Like attempting to stretch and relax a spring that is already under considerable tension. For a normal degree of ventilation, much greater effort is needed. This "mismatch" contributes to the sensation of breathlessness and is another price paid for airway dilatation achieved by hyperinflation.

To gain some appreciation yourself of how important a factor this is in the perception of breathlessness try it! From a normal lung volume, take a breath in, about half way to full capacity. Then spend just a minute trying to breathe normally, at this hyper-inflated position. A minute will seem like a long time. Remember, those with airway obstruction are breathing at this high lung volume all the time.

Hypoxia

The link between hypoxia and breathlessness is weak. To the lay person, the reason we breathe is to take in oxygen. Whilst this is of course an important imperative, the first priority of the respiratory system is to maintain a normal pH. It is not possible to survive for long with a pH outside of the normal range. Control is achieved by adjustments in pCO_2 (pH and pCO_2 are intimately linked). So, if for example a metabolic alkalosis were to arise (e.g., after vomiting), to correct the high pH, ventilation would be reduced and CO_2 would accumulate. By reducing ventilation however pO_2 would also fall. Fortunately (within limits) this has no detrimental effect. The level of oxygenation we normally maintain (pO_2 11–14 kPa) is far above what is required to sustain life, even in the long term. A modest fall in oxygenation would not normally be perceived by the individual as breathlessness and it would not, per se, drive up ventilation. Only at a much lower level (pO_2 around 8 kPa) does the center in the brain stem responsible for protecting us from hypoxia wake up and start to take action.

Prevalence of Breathlessness in Advanced Respiratory Diseases

Studies of symptom prevalence in advanced diseases show wide variation. This variation is dependent on the symptom, the disease, and the stage of the disease. A systematic review [3] reported the prevalence of breathlessness in cancer studies at 10–70 % (10,029 patients) and in advanced COPD studies at 90–95 % (372 patients). In one cancer study [4], the incidence of dyspnea was 84 % in lung cancer and the next most frequent was 58 % in lymphoma. In this study, they also assessed severity of breathlessness by a dyspnea score. The most severe dyspnea was observed in lung cancer.

Idiopathic pulmonary fibrosis (IPF) is characterized by dyspnea. Kozu et al. [5] studied 65 stable IPF patients and correlated their Medical Research Council (MRC) Dyspnoea Grade [6] with exercise capacity and lung function. The percentage of subjects in MRC Grades 2, 3, 4, and 5 was 25, 26, 26, and 23 %, respectively. The MRC Grade correlated positively with 6 minute walking distance (6MWD) and gas transfer (DLCO).

Assessment of the Breathless Patient

Apart from understanding the underlying cause for dyspnea, it is also important to assess the impact that the symptom has on the patient. This applies both to the individual practitioner managing a particular patient and also to the researcher investigating new interventions. Such assessments may include qualitative descriptors of the experience, quantitative measures of the symptom and its influence on quality of life and functional assessments such as exercise tests. It is obvious that the choice of application of these will depend on the status of the patient and his/her wishes. An extensive literature on assessment tools already exists [7, 8].

Attempts to identify the underlying cause of breathlessness by studying the words or phrases used to describe the experience have largely been unsuccessful [9]. Although there do seem to be clusters of descriptors in specific conditions, such as the inspiratory effort needed in COPD, their usefulness in the assessment of the breathless patient is limited.

Quantification of the symptom is better evidenced and more relevant [7]. The Medical Research Council Respiratory Symptoms Questionnaire (MRCD) [6] is well validated and simple to apply, and has been used for other respiratory conditions too [5]. Another simple scoring scale of severity is the Numerical Rating Scale (NRS) [10]. This is a scale from 0 to 10 (no breathlessness up to the worst possible).

Apart from the actual symptom, there are a number of other concomitant symptoms that the breathlessness patient may experience at the same time, such as fatigue, mood changes, and loss of control. These are captured in the Chronic Respiratory Disease Questionnaire (CRQ) [11]. In the CRQ, the patient chooses those situations most important in terms of impact of dyspnea on his/her life. The questionnaire may then be self or healthcare professional administered. Four domains are identified: dyspnea, fatigue, emotional, and mastery.

In the palliative context, it is rarely necessary to demonstrate or measure functional impairment objectively. If it is felt necessary, then exertional dyspnea can be simply assessed with the 6 Minute Walking Test (6MWT) [12]. Breathlessness at rest can be quantified by counting numbers [13]. This simple test involves the patient reading out aloud randomly generated two digit numbers over a 1 min period. From this the observer measures the total number of numbers and also the number of breaths taken. Thus the number of numbers per breath is calculated.

Management of the Breathless Patient

General Principles

The first stage after an assessment of the underlying cause of dyspnea will be to offer disease-modifying treatment in an attempt to reverse the process. Mostly this will be drug treatment, but, particularly in cancer-related dyspnea, radiotherapy or physical interventions may also be employed. These will be discussed in the lung cancer or mesothelioma chapters.

Purely symptomatic strategies for breathlessness management include:

1. Pharmacological management
2. Non-pharmacological management
3. Oxygen

Pharmacological Management of Dyspnea

Of the drugs that have been tried for the symptomatic relief of breathlessness, only benzodiazepines and opioids are widely used. Other drugs such as nebulized furosemide and antidepressants are unproven.

Opioids

The largest evidence base for drug treatment of dyspnea exists for opioids. A systematic review [14] described earlier studies. The conclusions were that there was evidence to support the use of oral and parenteral opioids, but not for the nebulized route. Most of the evidence came from studies in COPD patients, with less evidence for cancer and interstitial lung disease. Two more recent studies [15, 16] have explored the use of sustained release morphine and to define a starting dose. In the more recent study [16], it was reported that 10 mg sustained release oral morphine gave a beneficial response rate of 62 % which was not improved by dose incrementation. There were no episodes of respiratory depression in the 83 COPD patients involved in the study.

There are no studies looking at dosing of opioids for dyspnea in patients already taking them for pain.

Suggested Dosing Schedules for Opioids for Breathlessness

In opioid naïve patients, the options include a weak opioid such as codeine phosphate 15 mg 6 hourly as necessary, immediate release oral morphine suspension 1–2.5 mg

6 hourly as necessary, or modified release morphine, 10 mg once daily. Dose titration can be continued as for pain. The usual morphine side effects (constipation, initial drowsiness, and nausea) may well be encountered. Parenteral opioids are usually reserved for the end of life when the oral route is not appropriate. If the dose is started low and escalation appropriate, then respiratory depression should not be a problem in stable COPD, but intercurrent infection or other causes of exacerbations may interfere with this.

In patients already on morphine for pain, it is conventional to use short acting morphine at the appropriate rescue dose for dyspnea as well. Towards the end of life, the equivalent subcutaneous dose is used.

Benzodiazepines

The use of benzodiazepines for the palliation of dyspnea is widespread. A Cochrane Review [17] describes the 7 studies involving 200 patients with COPD and advanced cancer. They performed a meta-analysis of 6 studies and concluded that there was no evidence for the beneficial effect of these drugs for breathlessness in these conditions. They noted that whilst drowsiness occurred, it was less than with morphine. The drugs used were alprazolam (2 studies), diazepam (25 mg daily – 1 study), midazolam (8 and 20 mg daily versus morphine – 2 studies), lorazepam 1 mg daily (1 study), and chlorazepate 7.5 mg daily (1 study). They concluded: "These results justify considering benzodiazepines as a second or third-line treatment within an individual therapeutic trial, when opioids and non-pharmacological measures have to control breathlessness."

Suggested dosing schedules are listed below:

1. Stable COPD, where rest dyspnea is causing distress daily: diazepam 2 mg once daily.
2. Dyspnea associated with panic, requiring rapid palliation: lorazepam; 500 micrograms sublingually 6 hourly as required.
3. End of life respiratory palliation: midazolam 5 mg/24 h CSCI titrated upward as necessary.

Non-pharmacological Management of Breathlessness

Introduction

Non-pharmacological strategies are very varied in nature. Some are techniques are taught by the professional to encourage self-management by the patient, for example breathing retraining. Others require direct input from the therapist, such as acupuncture. A third group are those where a piece of equipment provides the therapy, such as handheld fans, which are self-administered, or applied by the practitioner, such as chest wall vibration. The other variable is whether the intervention involves an exercise component. The non-exercise interventions are well evaluated in a Cochrane Review from 2009 [18]. In this review, they are grouped as single (stand alone) or multi-component.

Single Component Interventions

These include acupuncture, distraction with music, and relaxation with prerecorded tapes, which includes progressive muscle relaxation. Although these are widely used in the palliative care setting, the evidence for their efficacy is limited.

The use and benefit of walking aids as are prescribed by physiotherapists have been studied in COPD patients. These include walking sticks, frames, wheeled walkers, or a vehicle to carry things. Four out of six studies showed significant improvements in breathlessness.

Two more complex interventions are chest wall vibration (CWV) and neuromuscular electrical stimulation (NMES). CWV involves the application of vibrators bilaterally to the chest wall or an inflatable vest connected to an air pulse generator for 3–5 min. It was concluded that there was evidence of benefit in the COPD patients studied, but not those with motor neurone disease [18]. The problem with this approach is the complexity of the technique, the need for expensive equipment, and lack of evidence of longer term benefit. In NMES, a portable NME stimulator is applied to the leg muscles (quadriceps, hamstring, and calf) and they are stimulated for 15–30 min/day for 3–5 days/week for 6 weeks. The studies demonstrated an improvement in quadriceps strength, symptoms, and walking distance in the COPD patients included at the end of the treatment period. The intervention was well tolerated. Whether NMES is a practical option for those patients unable to undertake conventional exercise programmes as in pulmonary rehabilitation remains to be seen.

The beneficial effect of cool air blowing across the face has been known to COPD and other breathless patients for a long time. The mechanism is thought to be stimulation of the nasal and oral mucosa by cold air. Many patients will describe the need to stand by an open window or door or have discovered the benefit of fans themselves. A study with a handheld fan held close to the face [19] showed a significant improvement in breathlessness as measured by a visual analogue scale over control (fan directed at the leg). The authors state: "The use of a handheld fan is an inexpensive, non-invasive, patient-directed, safe, practical technique for managing breathlessness in any setting."

Multi-component Interventions

Multi-component interventions can be subdivided into those that contain an exercise component and those that do not. The best documented example of the former is pulmonary rehabilitation, which is a central component in the management of

COPD. Exercise programmes have also been used in other chronic lung diseases and chronic heart disease. Although exercise is not a component of the type of multi-component intervention described by Corner [20], there is no reason why patients with cancer-related dyspnea who are able to undertake the type of exercise in pulmonary rehabilitation should not do so.

Multi-component Interventions: Without Exercise

The interventions included in these programmes are listed below. Different programmes will include different combinations of them [18]. The supervision may be by a nurse, physiotherapist, or multi-professional.

- Assessment involves understanding the cause of the breathlessness and the factors that make it better or worse.
- Counseling and support is difficult to define. It should include attention to physical and emotional issues, advice may be verbal or written. The interaction may be in the clinic or the patient's home.
- Breathing retraining encourages diaphragmatic breathing and other techniques to ensure breathing at a lower functional residual capacity (more efficient).
- Energy conservation, goal setting, and lifestyle adaptation.
- Relaxation and stress management.
- Psychotherapy.

Corner's programme was nurse led and included weekly sessions over 3–6 weeks. Sessions included counseling, breathing retraining, relaxation and coping and adaptation strategies. Twenty lung cancer patients were randomized to either receive the programme or follow up as a control group. There were improvements in median scores for breathlessness, distress due to breathlessness, functional capacity, and ability to perform activities of daily living in the treatment group compared with the control. These improvements were seen at 4 and 12 weeks after entry to the study. No improvement in anxiety or depression was seen. This led to a multi-center study of a similar nurse led intervention [21]. One-hundred and nineteen patients were randomized, there were significant improvements at 8 weeks in breathlessness at best, WHO performance status, levels of depression and distress and breathlessness from the Rotterdam symptom checklist.

These early studies of Corner [20] and Bredin [21] have led to the development of multi-component lung cancer dyspnea programmes in many centers. It has been observed however that not all patients need all of the components of the programme [22]. It is suggested therefore that the programme needs to be tailored to the individual and his/her needs.

One of the problems of such studies is that most of the patients have a poor prognosis and many symptoms will be deteriorating from week to week so there will be a considerable dropout rate, making quantitative assessment of benefit difficult. An alternative approach is a qualitative assessment by semi-structured interview and analysis of common key themes. Wood [23] performed such a study in 9 patients with advanced intrathoracic malignancy (6 mesothelioma and 3 lung cancer). The major themes identified were:

1. Recognition of need but mixed expectations
2. A personally tailored programme
3. The personal touch and attributes of the therapist
4. Specific changes in coping achieved
5. The global impact of the programme
6. Difficulties and barriers to achieving change
7. Facing the uncertainties of the future beyond the programme

The improvements in breathing control and activity management along with the qualities of the therapist led to improved functional capacity, coping strategies, and self-control.

Pulmonary Rehabilitation

Pulmonary rehabilitation is "a multi-disciplinary programme of care for patients with chronic respiratory impairment that is individually tailored and designed to optimize each patient's physical and social performance and autonomy. It is widely used for patients with COPD" [24]. The programme will include incremental exercise (walking, treadmill, or cycle ergometer), arm and shoulder exercises, respiratory muscle training, breathing retraining, education, psychological and social support and nutritional advice [25]. Pulmonary rehabilitation can take place in a variety of settings such as inpatient, outpatients, or in the community. A meta-analysis [26] showed significant improvements in the dyspnea, mastery, fatigue, and emotional function domains of the CRQ. The authors conclude: "rehabilitation relieves dyspnoea and fatigue, improves emotional function and enhances patients' sense of control over their condition. These improvements are moderately large and clinically significant."

In summary, pulmonary rehabilitation is a well researched and documented intervention for the management of breathlessness in patients with chronic lung disease. It should be offered to all patients well enough to participate. More work needs to be done to assess the role of exercise in the management of cancer-related dyspnea.

Oxygen

Rational and safe use of oxygen is discussed in detail in the COPD chapter. However, oxygen is widely used in the palliative setting for the relief of dyspnea without an assessment of the oxygen saturation (SpO_2) or partial pressure of oxygen in arterial blood (PaO_2). In a double blind trial [27], Abernethy compared breathlessness, measured on a numerical rating scale, in dyspneic patients with chronic lung disease (predominantly COPD). They were randomized to receive either oxygen or air by nasal cannula at 2 l/min for at least 15 h/day for 7 days. Breathlessness scores were repeated morning and evening throughout. There was no difference in the symptomatic benefit reported between the two groups. The important fact was that the mean PaO_2 of the oxygen group was 10.3 and the air group, 10.1. In other words, the patients were not significantly hypoxemic. This confirms the long-held belief that supplemental oxygen does not benefit patients who are breathless but not hypoxic. In practice, we do not measure arterial blood gases, but rely on measuring SpO_2 by pulse oximetry. It is recommended oxygen is not offered to those patients whose SpO_2 is 90 % or greater.

Carers and Their Needs

Whilst dyspnea causes considerable physical and emotional distress to the patient, it also can have a significant impact on the carers. This has been the subject of a qualitative study of ten lung cancer patients and ten COPD patients and their carers [28]. The authors commented that the patients developed stoical, philosophical coping strategies for living with their symptoms. Carers, on the other hand, felt anxious, preoccupied, and helpless in their role and needed support. Mostly this came from their general practitioner, or in the case of COPD patients, the respiratory clinical nurse specialist.

Approach to the Breathless Patient

The next question is the timing of applying the various strategies for managing dyspnea that have been described. In general terms, the first step would be by treating the underlying cause (i.e., disease modification). If the patient is capable of it, then non-pharmacological interventions should be offered, including exercise-based programmes if feasible. When the patient is not capable of exertion, or is breathless at rest, pharmacological treatment becomes more relevant. The problem with both opioids and benzodiazepines is that while they reduce the symptom and its emotional concomitants, the sedating side effects tend to reduce the desire for physical activity. Many components of the non-exercise programmes are relevant at this time too. These include breathing control, energy conservation, stress management and relaxation as well as use of fans. Oxygen may also be relevant.

As the end of life approaches, there will be increasing reliance on drug treatment with opioids and benzodiazepines, but fans may also still be relevant. Table 2.2 summarizes an approach to dyspnea management.

The recent American Thoracic Society statement on dyspnea [29] stresses the importance of detecting and relieving the underlying cause first, then if possible addressing associated cardiovascular deconditioning (with exercise) before the physical and pharmacological interventions described above.

Table 2.2 Outline of breathlessness management

1. Identify mechanism and cause
2. Treat (modify) underlying disease process as appropriate. This should be continued throughout until it is felt to be inappropriate
3. Check SpO$_2$ at rest and exertion if relevant
4. Exertion related dyspnea: consider exercise-based programme such as pulmonary rehabilitation
5. Exertion-related dyspnea: unable to do exercise programme, consider: non-pharmacological multi-component programme, not all components of the programme may be needed
6. Other options for exertional dyspnea:
   Walking aids
   Hand held fan
   Ambulatory oxygen if SpO$_2$ drops below 90 % on exertion
   Diazepam 2 mg once daily
   Codeine phosphate 15 mg twice daily
7. Rest dyspnea, but stable
   Non-pharmacological multi-component programme, or parts of it
   Fan: static or hand held
   Oxygen if SpO$_2$ less than 90 %
   Escalating opioids and/or benzodiazepines as previously described
8. End of life
   Fan
   Oxygen if SpO$_2$ less than 90 %
   Sublingual lorazepam or subcutaneous midazolam
   Subcutaneous opioids

Breathlessness as a Prognosticator

One of the key components of the Gold Standards Framework is the identification of patients in the last 6–12 months of their life so that their palliative care needs can be identified and met, and indeed prognostic indicator guidance has been published [30]. Of the commoner respiratory diseases, COPD has proved one of the most difficult to predict. The severity of dyspnea is one of the components of most assessment tools [30, 31]. Sadly, the end of life trajectory for COPD is unpredictable and these tools are of limited practical use. Even when combined with other independent predictors of survival (body mass index, FEV1, and exercise capacity), patients in the lowest quartile had a median survival of over 3 years [31].

In cancer, a systematic review [32] identified a number of independent predictors of reduced survival in a total of 7,089 patients. These were poor performance status, cognitive impairment, weight loss, dysphagia, anorexia, and dyspnea. The median survival of the patients in these studies ranged between 1.8 and 11 weeks.

The Liverpool Care Pathway (LCP) [33] identifies dyspnea as one of the potentially troublesome symptoms at the end of life. Despite this, clinical experience suggests that as death approaches the symptom becomes less troublesome. This observation was confirmed in study of the prevalence of dyspnea in patients dying from cancer [34]. They found that as death approached the prevalence fell from 39 % at referral to the palliative care team to 23 % in the last week of life.

In summary, in chronic lung disease, whilst there is some correlation between severity of dyspnea and survival, its presence or severity cannot usefully be used to determine the approach of the end of life. However, palliation of a symptom should not be limited to the last year of life anyway.

References

1. American Thoracic Society. Dyspnea, mechanisms, assessment and management: a consensus statement. Am J Respir Crit Care Med. 1999;159:321–40.
2. El-Manshawi A, Killian KJ, Summers E, Jones NL. Breathlessness during exercise with and without resistive loading. J Appl Physiol. 1986;61:896–905.
3. Solano JP, Gomes B, Higginson IJ. A comparison of symptom prevalence in far advanced cancer, AIDS, heart disease, chronic obstructive pulmonary disease and renal disease. J Pain Symptom Manage. 2006;31:58–69.
4. Dudgeon DJ, Kristjanson L, Sloan JA, Lertzman M, Clement K. Dyspnea in cancer patients: prevalence and associated factors. J Pain Symptom Manage. 2001;21:95–102.
5. Kozu R, Jenkins S, Senjyu H. Characteristics and disability in individuals with idiopathic pulmonary fibrosis (IPF) stratified by medical research council (MRC) dyspnoea grade. Respirology. 2011;16:1323–9.
6. Fairburn AJ, Wood CH, Fletcher CM. Variability in answers to a questionnaire on respiratory symptoms. Br J Prev Soc Med. 1959;13:175–93.
7. Dorman S, Jolley C, Abernethy A, et al. Researching breathlessness in palliative care: consensus statement of the National Cancer Research Institute Palliative Care Breathlessness Subgroup. Palliat Med. 2009;23:213–27.
8. Mahler D. Mechanisms and measurement of dyspnea in chronic obstructive pulmonary disease. Proc Am Thorac Soc. 2006;3:234–8.
9. Wilcock A, Crosby V, Hughes A, et al. Descriptors of breathlessness in patients with cancer and other cardiorespiratory diseases. J Pain Symptom Manage. 2002;23:182–9.
10. Gift AG, Narsavage G. Validity of the numeric rating scale as a measure of dyspnea. Am J Crit Care. 1998;7:200–4.
11. Guyatt GH, Berman LB, Townsend M, Pugsley SO, Chambers LW. A measure of quality of life for clinical trials in chronic lung disease. Thorax. 1987;42:773–8.
12. American Thoracic Society. ATS statement: guidelines for six-minute walk test. Am J Respir Crit Care Med. 2002;166:111–7.
13. Wilcock A, Crosby D, Clarke D, Corcoran R, Tattersfield A. Reading numbers aloud – a measure of the limiting effect of breathlessness in patients with cancer. Thorax. 1999;54:1099–103.
14. Jennings A-L, Davies AN, Higgins JPT, Gibbs JSR, Broadley KE. A systematic review of the use of opioids in the management of dyspnoea. Thorax. 2002;57:939–44.
15. Abernethy AP, Currow DC, Frith P, et al. Randomised, double blind, placebo controlled crossover trial of sustained release morphine for the management of refractory dyspnoea. BMJ. 2003;327:523–6.
16. Currow DC, McDonald C, Oaten S, et al. Once daily opioids for chronic dyspnea: a dose increment and pharmacovigilance study. J Pain Symptom Manage. 2011;42:388–99.
17. Simon ST, Higginson IJ, Booth S, Harding R, Bausewein C. Benzodiazepines for the relief of breathlessness in advanced disease in adults. Cochrane Database Syst Rev. 2010;(1). DOI:10.1002/14652858.CD007354.pub2.

18. Bausewein C, Booth S, Gysels M, Higginson IJ. Non-pharmacological interventions for breathlessness in advanced stages of malignant and non-malignant diseases (review). The Cochrane Library 2009;(3). DOI:10.1002/14651858.CD005623.pub2.
19. Galbraith S, Fagan P, Perkins P, Lynch A, Booth S. Does the use of a handheld fan improve chronic dyspnea? A randomised controlled, crossover trial. J Pain Symptom Manage. 2010;39:831–8.
20. Corner J, Plant H, A'Hern R, Bailey C. Non-pharmacological intervention for breathlessness in lung cancer. Palliat Med. 1996;10:299–305.
21. Bredin M, Corner J, Krishnasamy M, et al. Multicentre randomised controlled trial of nursing intervention for breathlessness in patients with lung cancer. Br Med J. 1999;318:901–4.
22. Connors S, Graham S, Peel T. An evaluation of a physiotherapy-led non-pharmacological breathlessness programme for patients with intrathoracic malignancy. Palliat Med. 2007;21: 285–7.
23. Wood H, Connors S, Dogan S, Peel T. Individual experiences and impacts of a physiotherapist-led, non-pharmacological, breathlessness programme for patients with intrathoracic malignancy – a qualitative study. Palliat Med. 2012. doi:10.177/0269216312464093. Accessed 5 Nov 2012.
24. British Thoracic Society Standards of Care Subcommittee on Pulmonary Rehabilitation. Pulmonary rehabilitation. Thorax. 2001;56:827–34.
25. Donner CF, Muir JF. Rehabilitation and Chronic Care Scientific Group of the European Respiratory Society. Selection criteria and programmes for pulmonary rehabilitation in COPD patients. Eur Respir J. 1997;10:744–57.
26. Lacasse Y, Goldstein R, Lasserson TJ, Martin S. Pulmonary rehabilitation for chronic obstructive pulmonary disease. Cochrane Review. 2009; Cochrane Collaboration. DOI:10.1002/16511858.CD003793.pub2.
27. Abernethy AP, McDonald CF, Frith PA, et al. Effect of palliative oxygen versus room air in relief of breathlessness in patients with refractory dyspnoea: a double–blind, randomised controlled trial. Lancet. 2010;376:784–93.
28. Booth S, Silvester S, Todd C. Breathlessness in cancer and chronic obstructive pulmonary disease: using a qualitative approach to describe the experience of patients and carers. Palliat Support Care. 2003;1:337–44.
29. Pashall MB, Schwartzstein RM, Adams L, et al. An official American Thoracic Society Statement: update on the mechanisms, assessment, and management of dyspnea. Am J Respir Crit Care Med. 2012;185:432–52.
30. Prognostic Indicator Guidance (PIG). 4th ed. 2011. www.goldstandardsframework.org.uk. Accessed 1 Apr 2012.
31. Celli BR, Cote CG, Marin JM, et al. The Body-mass index, airflow Obstruction, Dyspnea, and Exercise capacity (BODE) index in chronic obstructive pulmonary disease. N Engl J Med. 2004;350:1005–11.
32. Vigano A, Dorgan M, Buckingham J, et al. Survival prediction in terminal cancer patients: a systematic review of the medical literature. Palliat Med. 2000;14:363–74.
33. Marie Curie Palliative Care Institute. Liverpool care pathway for the dying patient. 2009. http://www.liv.ac.uk/mcpcil/liverpool-care-pathway/. Accessed 1 Apr 2012.
34. Edmonds P, Higginson I, Altmann D, Sen-gupta G, McDonnell M. Is the presence of dyspnea a risk factor for morbidity in cancer patients? J Pain Symptom Manage. 2000;19:15–22.

Chapter 3
Hemoptysis

Bernard Higgins

Abstract Hemoptysis is an alarming symptom which is distressing for patients and their families. Where possible it is best treated by addressing the underlying cause. Radiotherapy is usually effective in controlling hemoptysis from a bronchial carcinoma, for example. Massive hemoptysis is defined as >200 mls in 24 h. When a major vessel is eroded, bleeding may be catastrophic and rapidly fatal, and there is little to be done except to ensure that the patient is given medications such as benzodiazepines and opioids to relieve anxiety and breathlessness. If the patient survives, the initial bleed resuscitation is directed at maintaining the airway and circulatory volume. Most major bleeding arises from the bronchial arteries and bronchial artery embolization is usually effective in stopping bleeding by occluding the vascular supply.

Keywords Hemoptysis • Massive hemoptysis • Radiotherapy • Brachytherapy Bronchial artery embolization

Hemoptysis is an alarming symptom, and one which usually prompts the patient to seek medical attention. The majority of cases which a health care professional sees will therefore tend to be of small volume hemoptysis and, while investigation to determine the cause is clearly appropriate, the symptom itself does not usually require immediate treatment other than reassurance.

This is not always the case. Some people find hemoptysis distressing even if the volume of blood loss is small. Furthermore, in a small but important number of cases, bleeding from intrapulmonary lesions can be more substantial. It is not possible to define a precise cut-off point at which hemoptysis definitely requires treatment since this depends on several factors including the respiratory and circulatory

B. Higgins, MB ChB (Hons), M.D.
Department of Respiratory Medicine, Freeman Hospital,
Freeman Road, Newcastle upon Tyne NE7 7DN, UK
e-mail: b.g.higgins@ncl.ac.uk

S.J. Bourke, E.T. Peel (eds.), *Integrated Palliative Care of Respiratory Disease*,
DOI 10.1007/978-1-4471-2230-2_3, © Springer-Verlag London 2013

response of the patient, but the volume of blood loss may itself suggest a need for action. There is no universally accepted definition of major or massive hemoptysis, but many articles refer to a volume of >200 ml in 24 h. At this level, treatment of the symptom in its own right is clearly appropriate.

In general terms, hemoptysis is best treated by addressing the underlying cause. A huge variety of diseases can lead to hemoptysis. A small amount of blood in the sputum is not uncommon during the course of a simple respiratory tract infection, and other diseases which will be seen frequently in both primary care and by respiratory specialists will involve hemoptysis, including cardiac disease and bronchial carcinomas. However, hemoptysis can also be associated with a number of far less common conditions and the management of these varies hugely; for example, the approach to a patient bleeding from an arteriovenous malformation of the lung is very different to the management of a patient with diffuse alveolar hemorrhage secondary to a vasculitic disease. It is clearly outside the scope of this chapter to list all these situations, still less to attempt to cover their specific management. The focus here is on those situations where it is necessary, for palliative reasons, to control significant hemoptysis with direct treatment to its source.

Blood Supply to the Lung

The pulmonary circulation is well described and familiar to most doctors. The main pulmonary artery arises from the right ventricle and divides below the aortic arch into right and left branches. Each of these then divides into upper and lower branches, and thereafter further subdivision follows a much more variable pattern. There are a further 15–20 orders of branching before the vessels become pulmonary arterioles which ultimately break up into the pulmonary capillaries which envelope the alveoli. In health, and in most diseases causing hemoptysis, this is a low-pressure circulation in comparison to the systemic arteries arising from the left ventricle. The pulmonary artery pressure may, however, be elevated in the context of chronic hypoxic lung disease. It is estimated that only 5 % of clinically evident hemoptysis arises from the pulmonary circulation [1].

The commoner anatomical source of significant hemoptysis is the bronchial arterial circulation. The right and left bronchial arteries usually arise from the descending aorta just below the left subclavian artery. The commonest pattern sees two left-sided bronchial arteries and one common trunk on the right, but it is not unusual to find this situation in reverse, or a single stem on both sides, or two arteries on both sides [2]. Moreover, the arteries can originate further down the descending aorta. To add to this variation, in a minority of healthy people the bronchial supply arises from arteries other than the aorta; aberrant vessels might arise directly from intercostal arteries, the internal mammary artery, or the brachiocephalic or the left subclavian arteries.

In any of these cases, the bronchial arteries usually produce branches which follow the major airways with frequent smaller branches coming off the main vessels to create an anatomical vascular plexus in the adventitia of the bronchi, from which arterioles pass through the muscular layer and break up into capillaries in the submucosa. One particularly important aspect of the anatomical variation described above is that in some people the anterior spinal artery takes part of its supply from the bronchial arteries. This is important if clinicians are contemplating arresting bronchial bleeding by embolization of such a vessel since there is the risk of causing significant spinal cord damage. In a small number of cases, hemoptysis is from neither the bronchial nor the pulmonary circulation as delineated above. When hemoptysis is associated with a pulmonary sequestration, a totally aberrant arterial supply is to be expected. In addition, in cases of diffuse pulmonary hemorrhage, as in systemic vasculitis, blood loss is not associated with any particular anatomical site.

Management of Major Hemoptysis

Investigation

In the palliative setting, the cause of large volume bleeding will often be apparent since it is relatively unusual for massive hemoptysis to be the first presenting symptom in any disease process. When the relevant disease is known to be localized to a particular pulmonary lobe as, for example, in most lung tumors, management can move forward based on the reasonably safe assumption that the bleeding is from this site. However, in diseases such as bronchiectasis and cystic fibrosis where multiple areas of lung are involved, each of which may be the source of the hemoptysis, further investigation will be required to establish the site of bleeding. In the relatively small number of cases in which large volume hemoptysis is the first presenting feature, the most useful investigation is usually computed tomography (CT). A review of 208 consecutive cases showed that CT alone established a likely diagnosis in 67 % of cases [3]. The addition of fiberoptic bronchoscopy increased the yield to over 90 %.

CT and bronchoscopy will also be of benefit in cases with diffuse disease in which it is necessary to localize the site of bleeding. A CT scan will show alveolar filling in cases of significant bleeding, and this will usually be more obvious in one segment of lung than another indicating that this is the likely source. Profuse hemorrhage can lead to shadowing scattered over several segments, but this is less typical. Bronchoscopy can also localize bleeding to a degree and even if it does not pinpoint a source due to profuse bleeding and obscured vision, it is often possible to at least identify the side responsible which is important if a procedure such as embolization is being considered [4].

Treatment

The sections that follow this deal with specific treatment modalities which might be used in cases of major hemoptysis, but it is pertinent to consider also the small number of patients with a truly massive, life-threatening hemorrhage who require immediate resuscitation and stabilization. Such patients are relatively rare even in large referral centers, and because of this, and because of the virtual impossibility of conducting trials in such extremely ill people, there is little formal evidence on which to base advice. Indeed, even consensus guidance is difficult because each case has unique features, and because co-morbidity and overall prognosis determine what can, and what should be, done.

When a major blood vessel is eroded, bleeding may be catastrophic and rapidly fatal, and there is little to be done except to ensure that the patient is given medication such as benzodiazepines and opioids to relieve acute anxiety and breathlessness. If the patient survives the initial bleed, resuscitation is directed at maintaining the airway and circulatory volume. If there has been sufficient blood loss to produce hypotension, fluid resuscitation and blood transfusion may be appropriate. Because these cases are infrequent, we do not have the depth of experience available to our colleagues in gastrointestinal medicine who will see many patients with major upper gastrointestinal bleeding each year. Experience there is that overenthusiastic transfusion is deleterious and, while extrapolation from one disease system to another is not necessarily correct, it seems sensible to exercise similar caution in cases of hemoptysis. Administration of supplemental oxygen is sensible when required, aiming to treat to a target oxygenation value [5].

In centers with the available expertise, it may be possible to provide beneficial treatment via a rigid bronchoscope. Such centers will usually be those with cardiothoracic surgery on site. The technique of inserting iced cold saline into the segment responsible for blood loss with a bronchoscope inserted as tightly as possible into the segmental bronchial orifice has been described, as has the use of bronchial balloon tamponade [6, 7]. Balloon tamponade has also been described via a fiberoptic bronchoscope but the poorer direct vision and the relatively restricted aspiration abilities of the fiberoptic scope make this far less attractive, and generally speaking attempts to staunch bleeding via the fiberoptic bronchoscope are unlikely to succeed in a truly massive hemoptysis [8]. Where the relevant anesthetic expertise is available, it may also be possible to control bleeding, or to buy time by maintaining oxygenation, by using selective endotracheal intubation of the right or left main bronchus.

The ultimate treatment when all else fails is to remove the segment from which the bleeding emanates. This may be a suitable option in a patient with a good overall prognosis, but is rarely appropriate in the palliative care setting of advanced lung disease. The majority of patients presenting with massive hemoptysis will not be suitable for such invasive management. A treatment decision in this group of patients will clearly be easier when the person is previously known to the clinical team, but in all cases it is important at as early a stage as possible to agree what ceiling of care should be applied. In many cases, sedation with intravenous opiates or benzodiazepines is more appropriate than taking an aggressive surgical route.

Specific Therapy for Hemoptysis

Radiotherapy

External beam radiotherapy is long established as a useful mode of treatment in lung cancer. The overall value of radiotherapy in treatment of lung cancer is dealt with in Chap. 6. Most studies which have assessed the palliative benefits of radiotherapy have reported the combined benefit on a range of symptoms. However, where the individual response rate of specific symptoms has been given, hemoptysis is usually seen to be one of those which respond most readily. This has been the case in older studies such as the Medical Research Council study in 1991, and is still seen in more recent publications of large case series [9, 10]. It is not clear within these studies whether there is any systematic difference in response rates between tumor types, nor whether the initial severity of hemoptysis predicts the response. Intuitively one would expect cases with brisker bleeding to show benefit less readily, but moderately large volume hemoptysis can respond completely to a course of radiotherapy. Treating patients in whom hemoptysis is the predominant symptom has been shown to be of benefit in terms of improving overall quality of life [11].

Different radiotherapy regimens have been compared, although I am not aware of this having been done in a group of patients where hemoptysis is the main or only symptom. The generally accepted principle in palliative work for lung cancer is to aim for the fewest fractions possible since this appears to be no less beneficial, reduces the risks of adverse effects, and reduces the time that patients with a limited life expectancy need to spend on hospital visits [12]. Although radiotherapy is essentially employed as a treatment of malignant conditions, there are a small number of case reports of its use in other circumstances. Cases of hemoptysis due to mycetoma and mediastinal fibrosis have been treated successfully with radiotherapy [13–15]. Of note, these patients were described as having life-threatening hemoptysis, not simply small volume self-limiting bleeding.

Brachytherapy

The term "radiotherapy" is usually applied to radiation treatment administered via an external source. Treatment can also be given by positioning a radioactive source inside a body cavity close to the tumor, which in the case of the lung involves placing a source within the affected bronchus. This is known as intra-luminal radiotherapy or brachytherapy. Brachytherapy is carried out as part of an extended fiberoptic bronchoscopy procedure. Under light sedation a flexible catheter with a closed distal end is inserted through the biopsy channel of the bronchoscope, and is advanced across the area of tumor. A radio opaque marker is threaded down this catheter which is held in position whilst the bronchoscope is removed. A chest radiograph is then taken and the marker used to calculate the precise length of the catheter tube over which radiation can impact on the tumor. The marker is then withdrawn, and a small, highly radioactive source of iridium-192 welded to the end of a steel cable is passed down the catheter to deliver the radiation dose. It is shielded for most of its journey but is controlled by a computerized after-loader which exposes the source when it is in the appropriate position along the catheter. Because the strength of the source is known, its "dwell time" can be programmed over each 5 mm of the exposed area to allow precisely calculated doses of radiation to be delivered to the tumor.

There was initial hope that this elegant procedure might provide the benefits of radiotherapy treatment with fewer adverse effects. Unfortunately this does not seem to be the case. Although trials are not entirely consistent, external radiotherapy appears to provide better symptom control [16]. However, control of symptoms including hemoptysis can be achieved with brachytherapy, and one systematic review suggested that palliation with brachytherapy plus external beam treatment is superior to external beam radiation alone although this conclusion was not specific to hemoptysis [17]. Another reason that brachytherapy is not commonly employed is that there is a measurable incidence of massive hemoptysis, including fatality, after brachytherapy and probably caused by it. It is thought that this is mostly likely when the radioactive source has been lying directly against the bronchial mucosa or when an area close to a major blood vessel has been treated [18].

Because of these factors intra-luminal radiotherapy is not widely used in treating lung cancer but it does have one noteworthy advantage. Brachytherapy can be used in previously irradiated patients who have recurrence of symptoms including hemoptysis in situations where further conventional radiotherapy is not feasible because of dose thresholds. In one study of 270 patients with recurrent endobronchial disease after primary treatment, their response rate to brachytherapy for those with hemoptysis was 92 % [19]. Brachytherapy may therefore be of particular value in this "second line" role.

Bronchoscopic Therapy

There are a number of treatment modalities which can be deployed directly via a bronchoscope to treat hemoptysis when the symptom is caused by endobronchial disease. In general, these have been applied in the lung to malignant lesions, and their use has been restricted to a few centers. Bronchoscopically visible tumor causing hemoptysis has been successfully treated using the Nd:YAG laser (neodymium:yttrium aluminum garnet laser). An Australian study of 110 patients demonstrated beneficial effects on a number of symptoms, and once again the effect on hemoptysis was particularly marked with a 94 % response rate [20]. However, symptom response was generally better if laser therapy was combined with other forms of treatment. Coagulation using jets of ionized argon gas (argon plasma coagulation, APC) has also been described [21]. APC is widely used in gastrointestinal work to control bleeding lesions. Its disadvantage is that it can only treat to a depth of a few millimeters. Although cryotherapy has been used to treat bronchial tumors, I am not aware of any reported series in which it has been used for treatment for hemoptysis. There is no role for endobronchial stents in the control of hemoptysis.

Bronchial Artery Embolization

Whereas the techniques considered so far have involved attempts to stop bleeding via a bronchial approach, bronchial artery embolization attacks the problem by obstructing the vascular supply to the area of blood loss (Fig. 3.1). The procedure requires location of the bleeding vessel, and the variable origins of the bronchial arteries from the aorta can make this difficult, but an experienced operator can usually identify these reasonably swiftly. Once this has been done a bronchial arteriogram is performed. The expectation is not that this will allow direct visualization of bleeding with extravasation of contrast medium, as this is unusual. Rather, the operator hopes to identify an abnormal circulation such as a hypertrophied or tortuous vessel, or neovascularisation of an area, any of which implies that this is the likely source of bleeding. The confidence in this conclusion is enhanced by the prior radiological or bronchoscopic identification of the likely responsible area.

If the bronchial arteries have been identified and do not appear suspicious, a search must be made for another vascular supply. Whilst the bronchial arteries themselves can arise from sites other than the aorta, areas of lung disease can also acquire a separate systemic, non-bronchial blood supply. These feeder vessels may arise from various sites including intercostal arteries, the internal mammary, subclavian or even axillary arteries. Once an abnormal circulation has been identified, an embolic material

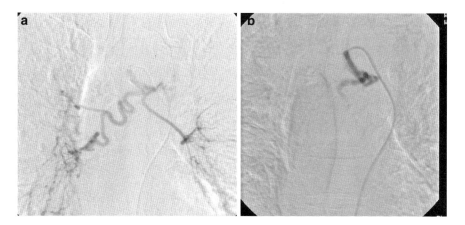

Fig. 3.1 Bronchial artery embolization. Bronchial arteriography showing an abnormal dilated bronchial artery (**a**) which was the source of massive hemoptysis. The bleeding was stopped by bronchial artery embolization which occluded the vessel (**b**)

is introduced via the catheter. Various materials are used including gelatine sponge, metal coils, liquid "glues" such as N-butyl cyanoacrylate, or polyvinyl alcohol particles. The choice will depend to some extent on the nature of the vessel to be occluded, but also to a large extent on the familiarity of the operator. There are no controlled comparisons of the available agents.

Several series have been published to demonstrate the effectiveness of embolization in managing major hemoptysis. The case-mix generally includes patients with cystic fibrosis, non-CF bronchiectasis, lung cancer (both primary and metastatic), aspergillomas and, in series from some countries, patients with active tuberculosis. The immediate success rate in those series reported in the past 2–3 years has varied from 72 to 100 % [22–25]. However, all these also report a substantial recurrence rate varying with the duration of follow up. For example, one Korean study of 108 patients, predominantly with non-malignant conditions, showed an immediate success rate of 97.2 % but a decline in freedom from recurrence over time; non-recurrence rates were 91.4 % at 1 month, 83.4 % at 1 year, and 56.8 % at 5 years [25]. Recurrence may be due to incomplete embolization, but more commonly to recanalization or to revascularization of the diseased area. The latter is more likely if the underlying disease cannot be controlled. This is an obvious problem in many cases of lung cancer, and series have also demonstrated poorer results in cases of aspergilloma [22–26].

Hemoptysis can occasionally be a major problem in patients with cystic fibrosis, and several reports have focused on this group. Unsurprisingly the occurrence of major hemoptysis is associated with more severe disease, with a high incidence of multidrug-resistant bacterial cultures [27, 28]. The success rate of initial embolization was over 90 % in these series, although some patients needed more than one procedure, perhaps because of a high rate of bleeding from non-bronchial systemic vessels [27]. However, recurrence rates are also high and the prognosis of these patients with massive hemoptysis, without intervention via lung transplantation, is poor [27, 29].

The success rate of embolization has also been reported in an exclusively onco-logical population most of whom had substantial blood loss (43 % of the group had over 300 ml blood loss in 24 h) [30]. Hemoptysis could be controlled in most; 89 % had either a cessation or a definite decrease in the degree of hemoptysis. However, the cohort had a poor overall prognosis with a 30 day mortality of 30 %.

Although immediate success rates from bronchial artery embolization are good, the procedure can have adverse effects. There may be bruising at the arterial puncture site. Chest pain is a common complication, presumed to be due to ischaemia of the chest wall because of involvement of the intercostal arterial supply; this is almost always short lived. Dysphagia has also been reported because of involvement of esophageal branches, and again it is transient and self-limiting. The complication of greatest concern is spinal cord ischemia. The incidence of this varies between series but is generally low [31]. Visualization of the anterior spinal artery at the preliminary arteriogram should preclude embolization of that vessel.

Antifibrinolytic Agents

Tranexamic acid is a synthetic derivative of lysine and acts as an antifibrinolytic by competitively inhibiting the activation of plasminogen to plasmin. It is used to treat menorrhagia and its efficacy in treating trauma victims has also been demonstrated. It is widely used in an attempt to reduce major hemoptysis, particularly whilst other measures are being organized. However, although this has been common practice for years, there is surprisingly little formal evidence of benefit. The only formal trial of which I am aware randomized 46 patients with hemoptysis of variable cause to either tranexamic acid or placebo and failed to demonstrate any benefit in terms of reducing blood loss or shortening the duration of hemoptysis [32]. However, this trial can be criticized in a number of ways, and in particular the patient group were atypical of those in whom tranexamic acid would usually be employed in that the degree of hemoptysis was modest in many of them. Moreover, in a significant proportion of those studied no underlying lung disease was identified (although investigation was not extensive).

Anecdotally most physicians who deal frequently with hemoptysis believe that tranexamic acid has a role and will remember patients whose hemoptysis has recurred and improved in timing with the cessation and reintroduction of tranexamic acid. One such case has been described in a patient with cystic fibrosis recurring after bronchial artery embolization [33]. Despite the lack of firm evidence the use of tranexamic acid can be recommended as a holding procedure in cases of major hemoptysis. The usual dose used is 1 g three times daily orally or 500 mg – 1 g by slow intravenous injection (over 5–10 min) three time daily or 25–50 mg/kg by intravenous infusion over 24 h. Etamsylate, 500 mg four times daily orally, is an alternative agent with an unknown mechanism of action, although it is believed to work by altering the permeability of the capillary wall and possibly by promoting platelet aggregation. There is even less evidence for its benefit in hemoptysis than there is for tranexamic acid.

Reversal of Abnormal Coagulation

Occasionally hemoptysis is caused or significantly exacerbated by abnormalities of the coagulation system. In the palliative care context this is not common, but will be seen in a proportion of patients who require treatment with warfarin for some other condition. In patients with persistent low or modest volume hemoptysis, the question of whether anticoagulation should be stopped will depend on an individual risk assessment which must take into account the reason for starting anticoagulation. When hemoptysis is more substantial, and certainly when life-threatening, it is undoubtedly appropriate to stop anticoagulation and even to consider the use of prothrombin complex concentrates. The use of fresh frozen plasma may also be appropriate.

Patients receiving chemotherapy may present with significant hemoptysis and low platelet counts. If bleeding cannot be controlled and platelet count is below 50 × 10^9/l, it may be necessary to offer platelet transfusion. Among the commonest pharmaceutical agents used by patients with hemoptysis is some form of antiplatelet therapy, such as aspirin or clopidogrel, since these are in widespread use for primary and secondary prevention of atherosclerotic diseases. Again, decisions about stopping these drugs are based on an individual assessment of risk. There are no clinical trials to guide the decision in patients with hemoptysis, although one interesting study in patients with upper gastrointestinal bleeding showed an increase in mortality if antiplatelet agents were stopped beyond the immediate period in which treatment to the bleeding source was carried out [34]. These patients were taking aspirin for secondary prevention of known cardiovascular disease. This is clearly indirect evidence, but it would be reasonable to stop antiplatelet agents briefly in cases of major hemoptysis and to restart them once the bleeding is controlled, where there is a good indication for their use.

References

1. Remy J, Remy-Jardin M, Voisin C. Endovascular management of bronchial bleeding. In: Butler J, editor. The bronchial circulation. New York: Dekker; 1992. p. 667–723.
2. Cauldwell EW, Siekert R, Liniger RE, Anson BJ. The bronchial arteries: an anatomic study of 105 human cadavers. Surg Gynecol Obstet. 1948;86:395–412.
3. Hirshberg B, Biven I, Glazer M, Kramer MR. Hemoptysis: etiology, evaluation and outcome in a tertiary referral hospital. Chest. 1997;112:440–4.
4. Hsiao EI, Kirsch CM, Kagawa FT, Wehner JH, Jensen WA, Baxter RB. Utility of fibre optic bronchoscopy before bronchial artery embolisation for massive hemoptysis. Am J Roentgenol. 2001;177:861–7.
5. O'Driscoll BR, Howard LS, Davison AG, British Thoracic Society. BTS guideline for emergency oxygen use in adult patients. Thorax. 2008;63 Suppl 6:1–68.
6. Conlan AA, Hurwitz SS. Management of massive haemoptysis with rigid bronchoscopy and cold saline lavage. Thorax. 1980;35:901–4.
7. Hiebert CA. Balloon catheter control of life-threatening haemoptysis. Chest. 1974;66:308–9.
8. Saw EC, Gottlieb LS, Yokoyama T, Lee BC. Flexible fibreoptic bronchoscopy and endobronchial tamponade in the management of massive hemoptysis. Chest. 1976;70:589–91.
9. The Medical Research Council Lung Cancer Working Party. Inoperable non small cell lung cancer: a medical research council randomised trial of palliative radiotherapy with 2 fractions or 10 fractions. Br J Cancer. 1991;63:265–70.
10. Reinfuss M, Mucha-Malecka A, Walasek T. Palliative thoracic radiotherapy in non small cell lung cancer. An analysis of 1250 patients. Palliation of symptoms, tolerance and toxicity. Lung Cancer. 2011;71:344–99.
11. Langendijk JA, ten Velde GP, Aaronson NK, de Jong JM, Muller MJ, Wouters EF. Quality of life after palliative radiotherapy in non small cell lung cancer: a prospective study. Int J Radiat Oncol Biol Phys. 2000;47:149–55.
12. Lester JF, Macbeth FR, Toy E, Coles B. Palliative radiotherapy regimens for non-small cell lung cancer. Cochrane Database Syst Rev. 2006;(4):CD002143.
13. Falkson C, Sur R, Pachella J. External beam radiotherapy: a treatment option for massive haemoptysis caused by mycetoma. Clin Oncol. 2002;14:233–5.

14. Gulliver S, Holt SG, Newman GH, Kingdon EJ. Radiotherapy for a pulmonary aspergilloma complicating p-ANCA positive small vessel vasculitis. J Infect. 2007;54:215–7.

15. Crossno PF, Loyd JE, Milstone AP. External-beam radiotherapy for massive hemoptysis complicating mediastinal fibrosis. South Med J. 2008;101:1056–8.

16. Cardona AF, Reveiz L, Ospina EG, Ospina V, Yepes A. Palliative endobronchial brachytherapy for non-small cell lung cancer. Cochrane Database Syst Rev. 2008;(2):CD004284.

17. Ung YC, Yu E, Falkson C, Haynes AE, Stys-norman D, Evans WA, Lung cancer Disease Site Group of Cancer Care Ontario Program in Evidence-based care. The role of high dose rate brachytherapy in the palliation of symptoms in patients with non small cell lung cancer: a systematic review. Brachytherapy. 2006;5:189–202.

18. Hara R, Itami J, Aruga T, et al. Risk factors for massive hemoptysis after endobronchial brachytherapy in patients with tracheobronchial malignancies. Cancer. 2001;92:2623–7.

19. Kubaszewska M, Skowronek J, Chichel A, Kanikowski M. The use of high dose rate endo-bronchial brachytherapy to palliate symptomatic recurrence of previously irradiated lung cancer. Neoplasma. 2008;55:239–45.

20. Han CC, Prasetyo D, Wright GM. Endobronchial palliation using Nd:Yag laser is associated with improved survival when combined with multi-modal adjuvant treatments. J Thorac Oncol. 2007;2:59–64.

21. Morice RC, Ece T, Ece F, Keus L. Endobronchial argon plasma coagulation for treatment of hemoptysis and neoplastic airway obstruction. Chest. 2001;119:781–7.

22. Chun JY, Belli AM. Immediate and long term outcomes of bronchial and non-bronchial systemic artery embolisation for the management of haemoptysis. Eur Radiol. 2010;20:558–65.

23. Dave BR, Sharma A, Kalva SP, Wicky S. Nine year single-center experience with transcatheter arterial embolisation for haemoptysis: medium-term outcomes. Vasc Endovascular Surg. 2011;45:258–68.

24. Daliri A, Probst NH, Jobst B, et al. Bronchial artery embolisation in patients with haemoptysis including follow up. Acta Radiol. 2011;52:143–7.

25. Yoo DH, Yoon CJ, Kang SG, Burke CT, Lee JH, Lee CT. Bronchial and non-bronchial systemic artery embolisation in patients with major hemoptysis: safety and efficacy of N-butyl cyanoacrylate. Am J Roentgenol. 2011;196:199–204.

26. van den Heuvel MM, Els Z, Koegelenberg CF, Naidu KM, Bolliger CT, Diacon AH. Risk factors for recurrence of hemoptysis following bronchial artery embolisation for life threatening hemoptysis. Int J Tuberc Lung Dis. 2007;11:909–14.

27. Brinson GM, Noone PG, Mauro MA, et al. Bronchial artery embolisation for the treatment of hemoptysis in patients with cystic fibrosis. Am J Respir Crit Care Med. 1998;157:1951–8.

28. Vidal V, Therasse E, Berthiaume Y, et al. Bronchial artery embolisation in adults with cystic fibrosis: impact on the clinical course and survival. J Vasc Interv Radiol. 2006;17:953–8.

29. Barben J, Robertson D, Olinsky A, Ditchfield M. Bronchial artery embolisation for haemoptysis in young patients with cystic fibrosis. Radiology. 2002;224:124–30.

30. Wang GR, Ensor J, Gupta S, Hicks ME, Tam AL. Bronchial artery embolisation for the management of hemoptysis in oncology patients: utility and prognostic factors. J Vasc Interv Radiol. 2009;20:722–9.

31. Yoon W, Kim JK, Kim YH, Chung TW, Kang HK. Bronchial and a non bronchial systemic artery embolisation for life threatening hemoptysis: a comprehensive review. Radiographics. 2002;22:1395–409.

32. Tscheikuna J, Chvaychoo B, Naruman C, Maranetra N. Tranexamic acid in patients with hemoptysis. J Med Assoc Thai. 2002;85:399–404.

33. Graff GR. Treatment of recurrent severe haemoptysis in cystic fibrosis with tranexamic acid. Respiration. 2001;68:91–4.

34. Sung JJ, Lau JY, Ching JY, et al. Continuation of low dose aspirin therapy in peptic ulcer bleeding; a randomised trial. Ann Intern Med. 2010;152:1–9.

Chapter 4
Cough and Respiratory Secretions

Stephen J. Bourke

Abstract Cough is both an important defense mechanism for the lungs and a troublesome symptom. Treatment is first directed at the underlying mechanisms giving rise to cough. Codeine or strong opioids can help to relieve cough although their use is limited by adverse effects such as sedation and constipation. Patients with ineffective cough due to neuromuscular diseases, such as motor neurone disease, are vulnerable to retained airway secretions and pneumonia. Physiotherapy techniques and cough assist devices may enhance clearance of respiratory secretions under these circumstances. Anticholinergic drugs such as hyoscine or glycopyrronium are effective in controlling secretions and a death rattle at the end of life.

Keywords Cough • Respiratory secretions • Hyoscine • Glycopyrronium • Chest physiotherapy • Cough assist devices • Death rattle

In palliative care, cough is both an important defense mechanism for the lungs and a troublesome symptom. Persistent cough has a substantial impact on health, daily activities, and quality of life, and can give rise to secondary symptoms such as retching, pain, headache, sleep disturbance, urinary incontinence, and exhaustion. Cough is also an important mechanism in clearing airway secretions. Failure to clear secretions causes a sensation of chest tightness and congestion, breathlessness and rattle, and predisposes to pneumonia and respiratory failure. Clearance of secretions may be impaired where there is ineffective cough, altered mucus characteristics, impaired mucociliary clearance, or structural lung damage. Each situation requires careful assessment and specific treatment targeted at the particular circumstances of the individual patient.

S.J. Bourke, M.D., FRCP, FRCPI, DCH
Department of Respiratory Medicine, Royal Victoria Infirmary,
Queen Victoria Road, Newcastle upon Tyne NE1 4LP, UK
e-mail: stephen.bourke@nuth.nhs.uk

S.J. Bourke, E.T. Peel (eds.), *Integrated Palliative Care of Respiratory Disease*,
DOI 10.1007/978-1-4471-2230-2_4, © Springer-Verlag London 2013

Mechanisms of Cough

Direct stimulation of the larynx provokes an immediate expiratory effort as an "expiration reflex," which acts to expel any inhaled foreign body. This reflex does not include an inspiratory phase which would tend to suck material into the lungs. In contrast, classic cough usually begins with an inspiratory phase before a forced expiratory maneuver, initially against a closed glottis, followed by expulsion of air on glottic opening [1, 2]. An effective cough generates a column of expired air moving rapidly through the bronchial tree dislodging mucus and material from the bronchial mucosa and propelling it outwards from the lungs. The first phase is a full inspiration to a high lung volume. The second is a compressive phase and this occurs when the glottis closes for about 0.2 s, during which there is contraction of the thoracic and abdominal muscles against a fixed diaphragm with rising intrathoracic and intra-abdominal pressure. The third phase is an expiratory phase with rapid expulsion of air when the glottis opens. During vigorous coughing, intrathoracic pressures of up to 300 mmHg and expiratory velocities of up to 500 miles per hour may be generated. Cough acts to clear the airway when there are large amounts of mucus due to excessive secretions or impaired mucociliary clearance. The removal of secretions is dependent on the shearing force produced by the air stream and the viscosity of the mucus. An ineffective cough predisposes to aspiration pneumonia and the accumulation of secretions in the airways can also cause breathlessness, rattle, and a sensation of chest tightness and congestion. The effectiveness of cough depends on several factors, including the patency of the airways, bronchial collapsibility, lung volumes, respiratory muscle strength, and the amount and viscosity of the mucus. Patients with neuromuscular disease, such as motor neurone disease or muscular dystrophy, who have inspiratory muscle weakness, will inhale only a small volume of air, but inspiratory muscle weakness must be severe before it affects cough. In contrast, expiratory muscle weakness may have a more profound effect as mild to moderate degrees of expiratory muscle weakness affect the expiratory pressures, airflow and cough effectiveness.

The anatomy and neurophysiology of cough are complex and incompletely understood. Studies have mainly been performed in animals and may not always be transferable to humans. Cough is usually triggered by physical and chemical stimuli which activate receptors in the upper and lower airways, pleura, pericardium, and esophagus [1]. The sensory impulses are then carried centrally to the brainstem via the vagus nerve. Motor impulses are transmitted to the effector muscles which include the diaphragm, abdominal, intercostals, back and laryngeal muscles. It is thought that rapidly adapting "stretch" receptors and C-fiber receptors are important, and recent research suggests that the type 1 vanilloid receptor may be the primary sensory mechanism in cough in humans [3]. Receptor responses can be augmented by inflammatory mediators, including histamine, prostaglandin E2, and cysteinyl leukotrienes. Angiotensin-converting enzyme inhibitor drugs, such as lisinopril, often increase cough sensitivity as they reduce the degradation of pro-tussive inflammatory mediators. Cortical input from higher centers can initiate or suppress cough. There may be different patterns of cough from different stimuli arising in different parts of the respiratory tract. A better understanding of the receptors and mechanisms involved in cough might lead to new improved treatments.

The compressive and expiratory phases of cough are a modified Valsalva maneuver and the high pressures generated can be transmitted throughout the body and give rise to additional problems such as urinary incontinence, rib fractures, musculoskeletal pain, pneumothorax, cough syncope, headaches, arterial hypotension, cardiac arrhythmias, and subconjunctival hemorrhage. Persistent coughing can be exhausting.

Cough in Lung Disease

Acute cough is one of the most common respiratory symptoms presenting to general practice [4]. It often occurs after an upper respiratory tract infection and is self-limiting and does not require treatment. Exclusion of more serious disease, such as pneumonia, and reassurance are all that is needed. Chronic cough can occur with almost any lung disease and assessment and management of the specific disease is essential. An isolated chronic cough in the absence of apparent intrinsic lung disease is most often attributed to gastro-esophageal reflux, rhinosinusitis and undiagnosed asthma or eosinophilic bronchitis. Chronic cough under these circumstances can be distressing and impact significantly on quality of life. Treatment is directed at the likely cause of the chronic cough with therapeutic trials of proton pump inhibitors for gastro-esophageal reflux, anti-histamines and nasal corticosteroid inhalers for rhinosinusitis, and inhaled corticosteroids for asthma or eosinophilic bronchitis. Sometimes a behavioral approach is helpful in suppressing the heightened cough reflex in patients with isolated chronic cough [5]. This involves education on the lack of physiological benefit of repeated coughing, strategies to suppress cough and the development of voluntary control over cough.

In the palliative care of advanced respiratory disease, cough is a common symptom but its significance may be masked by the dominance of other symptoms. In patients with lung cancer, a study of the pattern of symptoms and the efficacy of symptom relief showed that almost 80 % of patients had cough at presentation, and in half of these the cough was graded as moderate or severe [6]. Throughout the palliative course of the disease, cough persisted and was not fully suppressed by palliative treatments. In these patients, symptoms such as hemoptysis and chest pain were relatively well palliated whereas cough and breathlessness were more difficult to control.

Radiotherapy was particularly effective in improving cough in patients with endobronchial tumors where this treatment was appropriate. Bronchorrhea, in which there is hypersecretion of very large volumes of clear sputum, is a rare manifestation of mucinous bronchioloalveolar carcinoma (multifocal lepidic adenocarcinoma), and may respond to specific treatment with tyrosine kinase inhibitors such as geftinib or erlotinib [7]. Although breathlessness is the dominant symptom in patients with idiopathic pulmonary fibrosis, these patients often have cough with a markedly enhanced cough responsiveness to capsaicin challenge, although the precise mechanisms involved are uncertain [8]. Similar results are also found in patients with lung fibrosis due to systemic sclerosis [9]. Chronic cough is one of the most common symptoms in patients with chronic obstructive pulmonary disease (COPD), and these patients also have increased responsiveness to capsaicin challenge [10].

Chronic cough is an important symptom which has a substantial adverse effect on quality of life [11, 12]. It results in substantial physical and psychological morbidity. Quantitative assessment of cough in patients with cystic fibrosis using an ambulatory recording device showed that they had a median of 643 coughs per day (range 324–1,569). The cough rate was substantially higher when awake than when asleep [13].

Even though patients were studied in a stable phase, many had unremitting cough when awake, sometimes having more than 100 coughs per hour. This level of coughing is distressing for patients and has an adverse effect on their daily activities, social interactions, and quality of life. It makes them avoid theaters, cinemas, lecture theaters, and other situations where their cough is embarrassing and irritating to others.

Chronic cough gives rise to secondary symptoms such as headaches, retching, vomiting, musculoskeletal pain, sleep disturbance, exhaustion, and urinary incontinence. Depression is common in patients with chronic cough and improvements in cough with treatment correlates significantly with improvement in depression scores [14].

The mechanisms provoking cough in each of these diseases are very different and require a specific approach to treatment.

Clearance of Secretions (Table 4.1)

In the palliative care of many advanced respiratory diseases, clearance of airway secretions is an important aspect of treatment. This is particularly the case in patients with chronic suppurative lung diseases such as cystic fibrosis, diffuse bronchiectasis, and in some patients with advanced chronic obstructive pulmonary disease (COPD), where large volumes of sputum may overwhelm the mucociliary clearance mechanisms. Patients with ineffective cough due to neuromuscular diseases, such as motor neurone disease or muscular dystrophy, are particularly vulnerable to retained airway secretions and pneumonia. Cough suppressants are not usually appropriate in these patients, although they may be used at night in the palliative phases of the disease if cough is disturbing sleep.

In patients with copious sputum production and an effective cough, the initial approach is to reverse or ameliorate the cause by use of specific treatments. In patients with cystic fibrosis or diffuse bronchiectasis, a prolonged course of high-dose intravenous antibiotics is often the most effective measure in relieving symptoms even in end stage disease, and may remain an appropriate treatment even in patients approaching death [15, 16]. A number of mucolytic or mucokinetic drugs are used in specific diseases [17]. Nebulized 0.9 % sodium chloride is sometimes used in patients with COPD

Table 4.1 Non-drug interventions for cough

Airway clearance techniques
Forced expiratory technique ("huffing")
Autogenic drainage
Active cycle of breathing
Postural drainage
Positive expiratory pressure devices
Chest wall oscillation devices
Cough assistance techniques
Glossopharyngeal ("frog") breathing
Manual cough assist ("thrust")
In-exsufflation devices
Removal of secretions
Oropharyngeal suctioning
Patient positioning

or other lung diseases in an attempt to improve expectoration, although its effect is modest. Hypertonic 6–7 % sodium chloride has been shown to be effective in patients with cystic fibrosis and diffuse bronchiectasis of other causes [17, 18]. It improves hydration of the airway surface liquid and enhances sputum clearance but it can provoke coughing which may be distressing and exhausting for patients with advanced disease. Hypertonic sodium chloride sometimes provokes bronchospasm so that patients may benefit from prior use of a bronchodilator drug such as salbutamol or terbutaline. Inhaled mannitol also seems to improve mucociliary clearance in patients with bronchiectasis or cystic fibrosis [19]. It acts as an osmotic agent, drawing water into the airway mucosa. Dornase alfa (rhDNase) is widely used in all stages of cystic fibrosis but is not effective in bronchiectasis of other causes. The sputum of patients with cystic fibrosis is very viscous as a result of a high content of DNA derived from decaying neutrophils in the airway. DNase is an enzyme which cleaves this DNA thereby reducing the viscosity of the sputum making it easier to expectorate [17]. Stopping smoking improves the symptom of cough in patients with chronic bronchitis and COPD [20]. Carbocisteine is a mucolytic drug which has been shown to reduce the frequency of exacerbations in patients with COPD who have a chronic productive cough [21]. Inhaled anticholinergic drugs such as ipratropium or tiotropium may reduce mucus production although their effect on cough is not consistent.

In patients with suppurative lung disease, clearance of secretions can be enhanced by a variety of specialist physiotherapy techniques and devices [22]. Cough is the natural mechanism for airway clearance. However, in disease states, collapse of the airways may occur during the high intrathoracic pressure phase of coughing, impairing the clearance of secretions. The forced expiratory technique ("huffing") consists of forced expirations without closure of the glottis, starting from mid-lung to low-lung volumes. It can be particularly effective in patients with bronchiectasis or cystic fibrosis as an alternative to coughing. Patients can be taught the forced expiratory technique to enhance clearance without excessive effort. Physiotherapy is an integral part of the long-term management of these patients. Some techniques such as chest wall percussion and vibration require the assistance of a care giver while other techniques can be performed without assistance, giving patients independence in performing their own airway clearance. Autogenic drainage is a technique that uses controlled expiratory airflow during tidal breathing to mobilize secretions from the peripheral airways. The active cycle of breathing technique involves a cycle of breathing control, thoracic expansion exercises, and the forced expiratory technique. A number of mechanical devices can assist in sputum clearance. These include positive expiratory pressure (PEP) masks, and oscillating PEP devices such as flutter, Acapella® or cornet devices, as well as high-frequency chest wall oscillation vests [22]. The acceptability of airway clearance techniques is crucial and patient preference must be taken into account. The amount of time and effort involved can infringe on daily activities and can add to the overall burden of treatment in patients with advanced lung disease. Specialist physiotherapist input is invaluable in devising an airway clearance regimen that suits the individual patient's needs.

In patients with neuromuscular disease, cough becomes less effective as muscle weakness progresses. An effective cough requires a full inspiration, followed by glottic closure and adequate expiratory muscle strength to generate a high intrathoracic pressure and high peak expiratory flow. Physiotherapy techniques for improving the effectiveness of cough in clearing secretions are crucial in the management of these patients [23]. The inspiratory phase of cough normally fills the lungs to a high lung volume which optimizes the length-tension properties of the expiratory muscles and increases the lung elastic recoil pressure. In neuromuscular disease, a poor inspiratory effort results in only a small volume of air being inhaled.

Patients can be taught a glossopharyngeal breathing technique ("frog breathing") whereby the glottis sucks in air and then propels it into the lungs. Weakness of the expiratory muscles results in paradoxical outward motion of the abdomen with reduced expiratory flow during coughing. Manual compression of the upper abdomen and lower thorax ("manual thrust") can enhance cough flow rates and effectiveness. Mechanical means of assisting cough include insufflation-exsufflation devices. These deliver deep positive pressure insufflations followed immediately by application of a negative pressure to the airway opening during exsufflation. This enhances both the inspiratory phase of cough by increased lung inflation, and the expiratory phase by augmenting expiratory flow. Thus both manual and mechanical assisted coughing can enhance clearance of secretions [23].

Cough Suppressants (Table 4.2)

When a patient continues to have a distressing cough despite treatment of the underlying disease, the main pharmacological option is the use of opiates as a cough suppressant [24]. Codeine 15–30 mg 3–4 times daily is a weak opioid which has some cough suppressant effect [20, 25]. It is widely used in clinical practice but results are often disappointing and adverse effects such as constipation are common. Some studies in

Table 4.2 Drugs for cough and secretions

Cough enhancement

Nebulized 0.9 % sodium chloride 5 ml 4 times daily

Nebulized hypertonic (6–7 %) sodium chloride twice daily (bronchiectasis/cystic fibrosis)

Nebulized dornase alfa (rhDNase) 2.5 mg once daily (cystic fibrosis only)

Carbocisteine (capsules or suspension) 750 mg orally 3 times daily

Central cough suppressants

Codeine linctus 15 mg (5 ml) orally 4 times daily

Morphine oral solution 2.5–5 mg 4 hourly

Methadone linctus 2 mg (5 ml) orally 12 hourly

Peripheral cough suppressants

Simple linctus 5 ml orally 4 times daily

Removal of secretions

Hyoscine hydrobromide 150–300 micrograms orally 3 times daily

Hyoscine hydrobromide transdermal patch 1 mg/72 h

Death rattle

Hyoscine butylbromide

20 mg subcutaneously 4–8 hourly or subcutaneous infusion 60–120 mg/24 h

Hyoscine hydrobromide

400 micrograms 4–8 hourly subcutaneously or subcutaneous infusion 1.2–2.4 mg/24 h

Glycopyrronium bromide

200 micrograms subcutaneously 4 hourly or subcutaneous infusion 600–1,200 micrograms/24 h

patients with cough due to COPD or an acute respiratory tract infection show no benefit when codeine is compared to placebo [20]. Pholcodine 10 mg 3–4 times daily has similar efficacy but may be less constipating [20]. Strong opiates such as morphine, methadone, oxycodone, and fentanyl all suppress cough but their use is limited by adverse effects of sedation and constipation. A randomized double-blind placebo control study of morphine sulphate in patients with isolated chronic cough without apparent lung disease showed a significant benefit [26]. Patients were started on morphine sulphate 5 mg twice daily, and the dose was increased to 10 mg twice daily if cough control was not adequate. This low dose of morphine was effective in suppressing cough and was well tolerated. No patient had to discontinue treatment, although 40 % developed constipation and 25 % drowsiness, which was usually transient. Methadone is sometimes used to suppress cough at night because of its long duration of action but there is a risk of accumulation of the drug because of its long half-life. In the advanced stage of many respiratory diseases, patients may already be receiving opiates for other symptoms such as pain or breathlessness. Opiates act centrally in the brain stem in suppressing cough, although some studies in animals suggest that inhibition of peripheral cough receptors in the airways may also occur [27].

Many proprietary medicines are sold for the treatment of cough [28]. These contain a number of agents including demulcents, eucalyptus oil, maguisteine, benzonatate, and menthol, which may have a peripheral mechanism of action on cough receptors in the airways. Menthol has been shown to reduce cough in normal subjects undergoing a cough challenge study [29]. Benzonatate is chemically related to anesthetic agents and acts peripherally by anesthetizing the stretch receptors in the airways [30]. There are reports of its benefit in some patients but it is not licensed for use in the UK. Simple linctus 5 ml 3–4 times daily is a commonly used demulcent which some patients find soothing for a dry irritating cough. In general, the evidence of the effectiveness of proprietary medicines for cough is weak and they are not routinely recommended [28, 31]. In the palliative care of advanced stage disease, a number of other drugs have occasionally been used in an attempt to suppress intractable cough. These include dexamethasone, diazepam, gabapentin, baclofen, and nebulized lidocaine [32–34]. Experience of these medications is largely based on isolated reports in specific circumstances. Nebulized lidocaine may be effective in patients with severe cough near the end of life [33]. Baclofen has some cough suppressant properties acting centrally in the brainstem as a gamma-amino butyric acid agonist [34]. The current drug treatment of cough is very limited and there is a need to develop new agents. Specific vanilloid receptor 1 blocking drugs may be an area for future development [3, 4].

Death Rattle

Death rattle is the noise made by breathing through accumulated airway secretions in the dying patient. It is usually a sign that death is imminent. It is distressing for those at the bedside and possibly also for the patient. It is caused by retention of airway secretions in patients who are too weak to expectorate or who are unable to swallow. Airway secretions are synthesized in the salivary glands and bronchial mucosa, which are innervated by cholinergic nerves. Gentle oropharyngeal suction can be useful but is often ineffective. Anti-cholinergic drugs which block muscarinic receptors are the mainstay of treatment [35]. These agents can cause dryness of the mouth, blurred vision, palpitations, constipation, urinary retention, confusion, and delirium. Hyoscine butylbromide or glycopyrronium are non-sedating and may be useful in the conscious patient. Hyoscine hydrobromide (scopolamine) 400 micrograms subcutaneously every 4–8 h is the most commonly used drug. It crosses the blood–brain barrier and usually has sedative effects although rarely paradoxical agitation can occur.

Cough is an important mechanism in clearing airway secretions. Treatment of cough and secretions needs to be targeted at the particular circumstances. Some mucolytic and mucokinetic drugs can enhance sputum clearance in some disease situations. Mechanical and manual techniques can be used to clear secretions and to assist cough. There are very few effective cough suppressant drugs and opiates are the main pharmacological treatment for cough suppression. Hyoscine is useful in controlling secretions at the end of life.

References

1. Canning BJ. Anatomy and neurophysiology of the cough reflex. ACCP evidence-based clinical practice guidelines. Chest. 2006;129:33s–47.
2. McCool FD. Global physiology and pathophysiology of cough. ACCP evidence-based clinical practice guidelines. Chest. 2006;129:48s–53.

3. Groneberg DA, Niimi A, Dinh T, et al. Increased expression of transient receptor potential vanilloid-1 in airway nerves of chronic cough. Am J Respir Crit Care Med. 2004;170:1276–80.
4. Morice AH, McGarvey L, Pavord I. Recommendations for the management of cough in adults. British Thoracic Society guidelines. Thorax. 2006;61 Suppl 1:i1–24.
5. Vertigan AE, Theodoros DG, Gibson PG, Winkworth AL. Efficacy of speech pathology management for chronic cough: a randomised placebo controlled trial of treatment efficacy. Thorax. 2006;61:1065–9.
6. Muers MF, Round CE. Palliation of symptoms in non-small cell lung cancer: a study by the Yorkshire regional cancer organisation thoracic group. Thorax. 1993;48:339–43.
7. Popat N, Raghavan N, McIvor RA. Severe bronchorrhea in a patient with bronchioloalveolar carcinoma. Chest. 2012;141:513–4.
8. Doherty MJ, Mister R, Pearson MG, Calverley PMA. Capsaicin induced cough in cryptogenic fibrosing alveolitis. Thorax. 2000;55:1028–32.
9. Lalloo UG, Lim S, DuBois R, Barnes PJ, Chung KF. Increased sensitivity of the cough reflex in progressive systemic sclerosis patients with interstitial lung disease. Eur Respir J. 1998;11: 702–5.
10. Doherty MJ, Mister R, Pearson MG, Calverley PMA. Capsaicin responsiveness and cough in asthma and chronic obstructive pulmonary disease. Thorax. 2000;55:643–9.
11. French CT, Irwin RS, Fletcher KE, Adams TM. Evaluation of a cough-specific quality-of-life questionnaire. Chest. 2002;121:1123–31.
12. Birring SS, Prudon B, Carr AJ, Singh SJ, Morgan MDL, Pavord ID. Development of a symptom specific health status measure for patients with chronic cough: Leicester cough questionnaire. Thorax. 2003;58:339–43.
13. Kerem E, Wilschanski M, Miller NL, et al. Ambulatory quantitative waking and sleeping cough assessment in patients with cystic fibrosis. J Cyst Fibros. 2011;10:193–200.
14. Dicpinigaitis PV, Tso R, Banauch G. Prevalence of depressive symptoms among patients with chronic cough. Chest. 2006;130:1839–43.
15. Wolter JM, Bowler SD, Nolan PJ, McCormack JG. Home intravenous therapy in cystic fibrosis: a prospective randomized trial examining clinical, quality of life and cost aspects. Eur Respir J. 1997;10:896–900.
16. Bourke SJ, Doe SJ, Gascoigne AD, et al. An integrated model of provision of palliative care to patients with cystic fibrosis. Palliat Med. 2009;23:512–7.
17. Rubin BK. Mucolytics, expectorants and mucokinetic medications. Respir Care. 2007;52: 859–65.
18. Elkins MR, Robinson M, Rose BR, et al. A controlled trial of longterm inhaled hypertonic saline in patients with cystic fibrosis. N Engl J Med. 2006;354:229–40.
19. Jaques A, Daviskas E, Turton JA, et al. Inhaled mannitol improves lung function in cystic fibrosis. Chest. 2008;133:1388–96.
20. Molassiotis A, Bryan G, Caress A, Bailey C, Smith J. Pharmacological and non-pharmacological interventions for cough in adults with respiratory and non-respiratory diseases: a systematic review of the literature. Respir Med. 2010;3:199–206.
21. National institute for health and clinical excellence. Chronic obstructive pulmonary disease. NICE; 2010. http://guidance.nice.org.uk/CG101/Guidance/pdf/English. Accessed 1 Apr 2012.
22. Bott J, Blumenthal S, Buxton M, et al. Concise BTS/ACPRC guidelines: physiotherapy management of the adult, medical, spontaneously breathing patient. British Thoracic Society. 2009. www.brit-thoracic.org.uk. Accessed 1 Apr 2012.
23. Ambrosino N, Carpene N, Gherardi M. Chronic respiratory care for neuromuscular diseases in adults. Eur Respir J. 2009;34:444–51.
24. Wee B, Browning J, Adams A, et al. Management of chronic cough in patients receiving palliative care: review of evidence and recommendations by a task group of the Association for Palliative Medicine of Great Britain and Ireland. Palliat Med 2012;26:780–7. doi:10.1177/0269216311423793 published online before print October 2011.
25. Smith J, Owen E, Earis J, Woodcock A. Effect of codeine on objective measurement of cough in chronic obstructive pulmonary disease. J Allergy Clin Immunol. 2006;117:831–5.

26. Morice A, Menon MS, Mulrennan SA, et al. Opiate therapy for chronic cough. Am J Respir Crit Care Med. 2007;175:312–5.
27. Karlsson JA, Lanner AS, Persson CG. Airway opioid receptors mediate inhibition of cough and reflex bronchoconctriction in guinea pigs. J Pharmacol Exp Ther. 1990;252:863–8.
28. Schroeder K, Fahey T. Systematic review of randomised controlled trials of over the counter medicines for acute cough in adults. BMJ. 2002;324:1–6.
29. Morice AH, Marshall AE, Higgins KS, Grattan TJ. Effect of inhaled menthol on citric acid induced cough in normal subjects. Thorax. 1994;49:1024–6.
30. Doona M, Walsh D. Benzonatate for opioid-resistant cough in advanced cancer. Palliat Med. 1997;12:55–8.
31. Ostroff C, Lee CE, McMeekin J. Unapproved prescription cough, cold and allergy drug products. Chest. 2011;140:295–300.
32. Estfan B, Walsh D. The cough from hell: diazepam for intractable cough in a patient with renal cell carcinoma. J Pain Symptom Manage. 2008;36:553–8.
33. Lingerfelt BM, Swainey CW, Smith TJ, Coyne PJ. Nebulized lidocaine for intractable cough near the end of life. J Support Oncol. 2007;5:301–2.
34. Dicpinigaitis PV, Dobkin JB, Rauf K, Aldrich TK. Inhibition of capsaicin-induced cough by the gamma-aminobutyric acid agonist baclofen. Br J Pharmacol. 2003;140:261–8.
35. Wildiers H, Dhaenekint C, Demeulenaere P, et al. Atropine, hyoscine butylbromide or scopolamine are equally effective for the treatment of death rattle in terminal care. J Pain Symptom Manage. 2009;38:124–33.

Chapter 5
Pain in Respiratory Disease

Eleanor Grogan

Abstract Pain may be classified as nociceptive or neuropathic and somatic or visceral. Neuropathic pain can be further subdivided into that due to nerve compression, nerve destruction or sympathetically maintained pain. The chapter describes the assessment and diagnosis of the cause of pain and the concepts of total pain and regular and breakthrough pain. Management starts with explanation and general non-drug measures. Disease modification runs alongside the use of non-opioid analgesics and then the WHO opioid ladder. Oral morphine is the main strong opioid used, but the indication for alternative drugs and routes is considered. Neuropathic pain usually requires the use of adjuvant analgesics. The role of other adjuvants in certain circumstances is described as well as the use of topical analgesics and anesthetic interventions.

Keywords Pain assessment • Nociceptive • Neuropathic • Opioid • Adjuvant analgesics WHO ladder

Pain is a common symptom in respiratory disease; it is distressing to patients and is not confined to those with cancer. Significant pain occurs in approximately one-third of patients with chronic obstructive pulmonary disease (COPD) and in a comparable proportion of patients with lung cancer [1–5]. It is known that pain from cancer is frequently undertreated and there is no reason to think that pain from other advanced lung disease is better managed [6, 7]. Pain is a complex symptom which is sometimes difficult to manage well. There may be many causes for a patient's pain which may or may not relate to their underlying respiratory illness. To optimize

E. Grogan, B.Sc., M.B.B.S., M.A., FRCP
Department of Palliative Care, Wansbeck General Hospital,
Woodhorn Lane, Ashington, Northumberland NE63 9JJ, UK
e-mail: eleanor.grogan@nhct.nhs.uk

S.J. Bourke, E.T. Peel (eds.), *Integrated Palliative Care of Respiratory Disease*,
DOI 10.1007/978-1-4471-2230-2_5, © Springer-Verlag London 2013

pain control, the causation and mechanisms of the pain need to be understood and a variety of pain-relieving options should be considered. Pain is not measurable, except in so much as the patient describes it. Pain is what the patient says hurts and there may be many contributing factors apart from physical reasons. This is the concept of total pain, where physical, psychological, social, and spiritual factors all contribute to a patient's pain.

Pain Classification

There are many different types of pain and patients often experience multiple pains simultaneously. In one study of patients with cancer, approximately one-third of patients reported one pain, a third two pains, and a third reported three or more, but not all patients with advanced cancer experience pain [8]. To be best able to manage a patient's pain requires the clinician to ask the patient if they have pain, how many pains they have, and then to work through each one in turn to understand the etiology and type of each pain. Only then can the appropriate analgesia be considered. Pain may arise directly from a cancer or other medical condition, be due to treatments which have damaged visceral, musculoskeletal or nervous tissue such as surgery or radiotherapy, or may be pain unrelated to the predominant diagnosis, for example pain from an osteoporotic vertebral fracture in a patient with advanced COPD who has had many courses of steroids.

Mechanisms of Pain

Usually pain occurs when the body receives a stimulus that is perceived as painful. An impulse is transmitted upward from the peripheries via the spinothalamic tract to the thalamus and on to the cerebral cortex (Fig. 5.1). The spinothalamic tract is an ascending pathway within the spinal cord which relays sensory information to the brain. There are different ascending pathways for different sensory modalities. The sensation of pain is transmitted along with temperature via the spinothalamic tract. The other main sensory modalities are proprioception and light touch which are transmitted via different ascending pathways. The spinothalamic tract crosses to the contralateral side of the spinal cord almost immediately as it enters it. The descending pathway from the brain is called the corticospinal tract and it relays motor instructions down from the brain.

An example of this at its simplest would be a person who stands on a nail. The painful impulse travels up the spinothalamic tract to the brain. The brain recognizes that this is painful and wants the person to move away from the nail, so sends an instruction down the corticospinal tract so that the person moves their foot away from the nail.

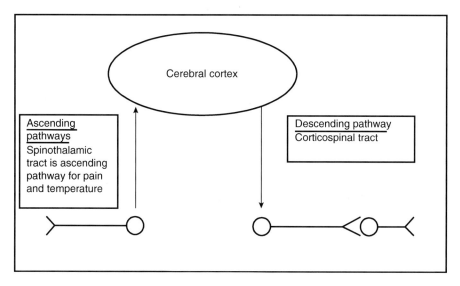

Fig. 5.1 Neurological pathways for pain. When the body receives a stimulus that is perceived as painful an impulse is transmitted upward from the peripheries via the spinothalamic tract to the thalamus and on to the cerebral cortex. The descending pathway is via the corticospinal tract

Patients with a disease process may experience pain without a painful stimulus because their disease has caused damage to the ascending pathways, nerves that feed in to the ascending pathways or nociceptors found on skin, bones, joints, and other parts of the body.

Example
Miss A. has lung cancer for which she has had a lobectomy. Since the surgery she has complained of persistent chest pain near her scar. She is experiencing pain not because of a painful stimulus, but because of damage to her sensory nerves by the surgery. This sends incorrect messages to her cerebral cortex via the ascending sensory pathways and so she experiences pain.

Types of Pain

Pain can either be functional (meaning normal pain that most people experience, such as tension headache) or organic (meaning pathological and related in some way to a disease process). Organic pains can either be nociceptive or neuropathic. Nociceptive pain is due to tissue damage, whereas neuropathic pain arises from damage or disease affecting the nervous system.

Nociceptive Pain

Nociceptors are sensory receptors at the nerve ending which are sensitive to noxious or potentially noxious stimuli. They respond to such stimuli by sending a signal via the spinothalamic tract to the brain. They are found in skin, bone, muscle, connective tissues, and thoracic, abdominal, and pelvic viscera. Pain is transmitted by both $A\delta$ and C-fibers, the latter being slower and unmyelinated. Pain transmitted through $A\delta$ fibers is felt as a sharp and immediate pain. Pain due to activity in the C-fibers is felt as a dull, aching sensation. Visceral pain is difficult to localize, whereas other nociceptive pain can often be well localized.

Visceral pain arises when the viscera are infiltrated, compressed, distended, or stretched by an underlying disease process. This pain is often described as a deep aching pain, is poorly localized, and can be referred to unusual sites: for example, patients with lung cancer and liver metastases with associated diaphragmatic irritation may experience shoulder pain.

Neuropathic Pain

Neuropathic pain results from injury to the peripheral or central nervous system. In patients with cancer, this is commonly due to compression or infiltration of part of the nervous system by the tumor. Compression generally precedes infiltration when directly due to cancer. It may be peripheral nerves, nerve roots or the spinal cord that are involved. Damage to each of these will give pain with differing characteristics. A study of over 200 cancer patients with neuropathic pain found that 79 % had nerve compression pain, 16 % nerve injury pain, and 5 % had sympathetically maintained pain [9].

Peripheral pain is more commonly seen than central neuropathic pain. As well as being directly related to disease, neuropathic pain may result from damage secondary to surgery (e.g., peripheral nerves in the skin being cut during surgery), chemotherapy, or radiotherapy. Drugs recognized as causing peripheral neuropathy include some of those used to treat tuberculosis as well as some of the commonly used cancer treatments [10–12].

Neuropathic pain differs in nature from other pains. Typically patients describe it as a background ache with superimposed shooting or stabbing pains. Neuropathic pain can be difficult for patients to describe – they may describe it as a sandpaper-like pain, a sensation of running water but painful or like an electric shock. In general, if a patient has an unpleasant pain that they are struggling to describe or pain in a numb area, it is likely to be neuropathic pain. Central neuropathic pain is less commonly seen than peripheral pain and may be due to damage within the cerebral cortex, brainstem or spinal cord, for example spinal cord compression.

Sympathetically maintained pain is pain arising from damage to sympathetic nerves. In addition to experiencing neuropathic pain, the patient also experiences symptoms associated with activation of the sympathetic nervous system such as sweating and redness of the affected area. It can arise due to malignancy within the thorax affecting the sympathetic nerves.

Total Pain

Many pains have obvious physical causes but some do not. Pain can be perceived as being worse by the patient when, for example, they are deprived of sleep or have psychological worries. Many factors can influence pain, both in positive and negative ways. The concept of "total pain" is when physical reasons are only one factor in causing the patient's pain. The other non-physical factors are just as valid as the physical factors, but the patient's pain will not be resolved unless the concept of total pain is addressed.

When asked to rate the severity of their pain, patients find that scores vary throughout the day. Pain can be perceived as being worse if patients are upset or agitated, if they are bored or depressed. Patients who are lacking in sleep often perceive their pain as being more severe, as will patients who do not understand what is happening to them. Conversely, patients may feel that their pain is decreased when they are relaxed and their mind is occupied by distractions (such as visitors, reading, or activities). Patients who accept what is happening to them, have relief of other symptoms, and are sleeping well often perceive their pain as being less severe. Total pain describes how social, spiritual, psychological, and physical problems interact to result in the experience of pain (Fig. 5.2). If the importance of the non-physical dimensions of the pain is not recognized, then the pain is unlikely to be adequately controlled despite analgesic medication.

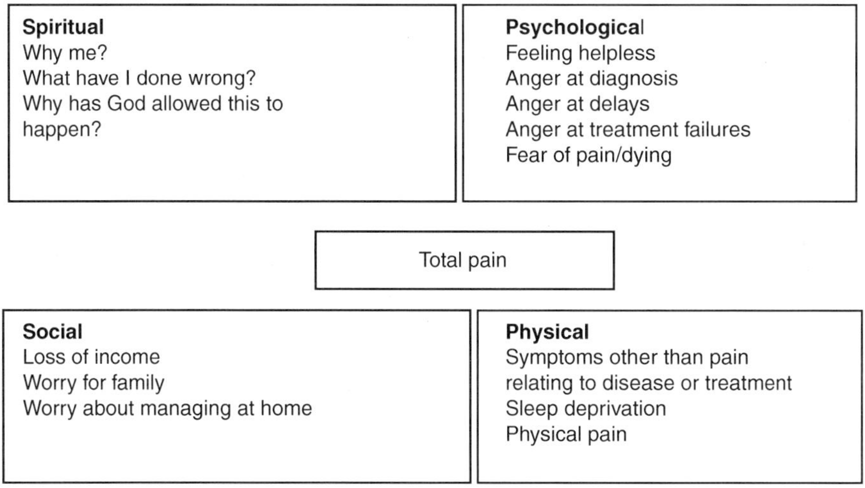

Spiritual Why me? What have I done wrong? Why has God allowed this to happen?	**Psychological** Feeling helpless Anger at diagnosis Anger at delays Anger at treatment failures Fear of pain/dying

Total pain

Social Loss of income Worry for family Worry about managing at home	**Physical** Symptoms other than pain relating to disease or treatment Sleep deprivation Physical pain

Fig. 5.2 Total pain: spiritual, psychological, social, and physical factors interact to result in the experience of pain

Regular and Breakthrough Pain

Not all pains are present all of the time. Pain that is present most of the time is termed "regular" or "background" pain and usually this requires regular analgesia. As well as this, many patients experience breakthrough or incident pain. This is pain that occurs despite regular analgesia. It is termed incident pain when it is predictable and breakthrough pain when it is not. Breakthrough pain can occur for no obvious reason but may be a source of distress to the patient. Patients may perceive this as a sign that their disease is worsening, but they should be reassured that this is not necessarily the case. Both breakthrough and incident pain require quick-acting analgesia. If the patient finds they are requiring several doses a day for breakthrough pain, this usually suggests that they are receiving inadequate regular analgesia.

Example
Mr B. has lung cancer with metastases in his pelvis. He is on morphine sulphate modified release tablets 10 mg twice daily and is pain free at rest. However, when he stands up he experiences a sudden severe pain in his pelvis radiating into his leg. As soon as he sits again, the pain resolves.

It may seem reasonable to increase his regular analgesia as he has required several rescue doses for his incident pain. However, this may well make him drowsy as he would effectively then have too much morphine in his system for the majority of the time when he is pain free. An alternative solution would need to be found whereby he just receives the extra analgesia when he needs it.

Example
Mrs C. has mesothelioma. She has had a constant painful ache over her biopsy site for several months. Since the addition of morphine sulphate modified release tablets 10 mg twice daily this had been well controlled. Recently, she has found that this pain has been coming back despite the morphine tablets. She has been taking morphine immediate release liquid with good effect, although it takes about 40 min to work. The pain recurs after a few hours. This pattern tends to happen three or four times a day. There are no obvious triggers for the flares of pain.

Mrs C's background analgesia is no longer adequate. Her background analgesia should therefore be increased. Although her pain may have changed, she should be reassured that it does not necessarily follow that her disease has worsened.

Pain Assessment

When assessing a patient's pain it is important to remember that pain is what the patient says it is. We all perceive pain in different ways and it is a multi-factorial symptom. Pain is often under-treated in patients with advanced disease. In the SUPPORT study, nearly 50 % of hospitalized patients reported pain and in a European study 56 % of patients reported moderate to severe pain from cancer, occurring at least monthly [13, 14]. Most patients with pain have more than one pain. It is therefore important not just to ask if they have pain, but instead to ask if they have pain and how many pains they have. The site of each pain then needs to be clarified and each pain addressed in turn. There are many mnemonics that can be used in the assessment of pain. One such mnemonic is SOCRATES [15]. This leads to comprehensive questioning about the patient's pain to ascertain how it affects the patient, the likely etiology, and the optimal treatment for that patient.

S site
O onset
C character
R radiation
A associated symptoms
T time course
E exacerbating/relieving factors
S severity

Diagnosing Pain

To treat any pain successfully requires accurate diagnosis. This may involve radiological imaging or other investigations, but it is also crucial to listen carefully to the patient's description. From this, it should be possible to determine the site of the patient's pain, whether it radiates anywhere, and whether it is neuropathic or nociceptive.

Example
Mr D has lung cancer. He describes having pain in his left shoulder. It radiates into his arm and sometimes down his arm. He is also aware of it under his arm. The pain is often severe and feels like a constant dull ache with bouts of burning or shooting pain. It is sometimes associated with weakness.

This is a description of neuropathic pain. It is likely that the pain is coming from his brachial plexus, and since there is some associated weakness, this is probably due to compression or invasion of the brachial plexus by his cancer.

As well as considering conventional analgesia for his pain it would be appropriate to commence a short course of steroids to reduce any tumor-associated oedema that may be exacerbating the pain and also to consider whether any specific anti-cancer treatment is appropriate.

Example
Miss E is admitted to hospital with a fever and right basal lung crepitations. Her chest radiograph confirms right basal shadowing consistent with pneumonia. Her main symptoms are that cough and chest pain. Her chest pain is sharp and worse on inspiration.
The cause of the pleuritic pain is inflammation of the pleura secondary to pneumonia.

Pain Management

Principles of Pain Management

There are many different types of pain and different classes of analgesic drugs. Not all types of analgesia work for all pains. The World Health Organisation's three step analgesic ladder has been used for many years as the method for initiating and titrating appropriate analgesia [16] (Fig. 5.3). A modified version is now available specifying the need to add, rather than replace, analgesia for nociceptive pain [17].

WHO Analgesic Ladder

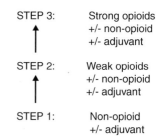

STEP 3: Strong opioids
+/- non-opioid
+/- adjuvant

STEP 2: Weak opioids
+/- non-opioid
+/- adjuvant

STEP 1: Non-opioid
+/- adjuvant

Fig. 5.3 World Health Organisation (WHO) ladder, outlining a step-wise approach to use of analgesics

Example

Mr F. has a new diagnosis of lung cancer. He is complaining of pain in his right anterior chest wall. He is awaiting an oncology multi-disciplinary team review as to what treatment he will receive. On further questioning using SOCRATES, he says that the pain started about 2 weeks ago and has gradually got worse. It is aching in nature and does not radiate. There are no associated features and he has taken the occasional paracetamol which reduces the severity from 5/10 to 3/10.

Mr F. needs regular, rather than just occasional analgesia. Taking regular paracetamol will provide more effective analgesia than he is currently receiving. Following the WHO pain ladder, if paracetamol alone does not provide adequate analgesia, it would be appropriate to add in a regular weak opioid or a non-steroidal anti-inflammatory drug.

Example

Mrs G. has ongoing pain from her mesothelioma. She is on both regular paracetamol and codeine phosphate. She finds that the severity of her pain was especially helped by the addition of ibuprofen. Her pain score reduced from 8/10 to 5/10. However, the pain still dominates her day. Her pain has not changed in nature and remains a constant aching pain.

Mrs G. is already on a weak opioid and a non-steroidal anti-inflammatory drug. Her pain seems to be visceral rather than neuropathic in nature. Following the WHO pain ladder, it would be appropriate to stop the weak opioid (codeine phosphate) and instead commence a regular strong opioid such as morphine sulphate modified release tablets.

Non-drug Treatment

Pain can be overwhelming, even when not severe. It can limit the patient's ability to perform activities and may preoccupy their life. They may find that all they can think about is their pain. It is therefore essential to manage a patient's pain by using non-drug methods as well as by using medication. Patients often need reassurance about their pain. They may worry that pain is an indication that their disease is worsening. This may be true, but will not be the case for all patients. To have an explanation of what is causing their pain or why it is worse is often helpful to patients. Sometimes there may be cultural beliefs associated with pain which the patient may be experiencing and they may benefit from talking these through. Careful discussion with the patient about their pain should be the first step to managing it. Having the right environment is critical to successfully managing a patient's pain. Imagine having persistent pain and being in the middle of a busy, noisy hospital environment where you are unable to sleep properly at night. You would be tired, less able to manage the pain, and may perceive the pain as more troublesome. If, on the other hand, you were in a quiet, calm environment where you were able to adequately rest and sleep and people were available to reassure you about your pain and listen to your fears, you may be likely to perceive it as less troublesome.

Because pain can be all-consuming, the patient may find it difficult to think of anything else. A useful pain management strategy is to provide a distraction to the pain, for example a project to do, someone to talk to, questions other than about their pain. Complementary therapies can also provide a distraction from the pain, as well as relaxing the patient and may provide some analgesic benefit [18]. It is thought that acupuncture may also provide some analgesic benefit to patients, but currently there is insufficient evidence to support this [19].

TENS (transcutaneous electrical nerve stimulation) is a further possible non-drug treatment that may provide some pain relief, although, again, there is little evidence to support it [20]. Electrode pads are applied to the patient's skin on either side of the painful area. They are connected to a machine that provides electrical stimulation to the skin. This in turn fools the brain into perceiving the pain differently. There are cautions and contraindications to using a TENS machine. In order to ensure safe use, it is essential that the TENS machine is initiated by someone who is knowledgeable and experienced in the safe use of this equipment.

Treating the underlying cause of the pain, if appropriate and possible, should always be considered. For example, if a patient has lung cancer with bone metastases and they sustain a pathological fracture, this will be painful. Treatments such as surgery or radiotherapy should be considered alongside analgesia as they may provide a more appropriate and lasting solution. Chemotherapy, radiotherapy, and surgery may all provide analgesic benefit to the patient, depending on the mechanism for their pain.

Non-opioid Analgesia

Paracetamol

Paracetamol is a centrally acting non-opioid analgesic. It blocks the enzyme cyclooxygenase (COX) and so inhibits the production of prostaglandins which are implicated in pain mechanisms [21]. There are two main iso-enzymes of COX which are expressed to varying levels by different tissues. COX-1 is produced constitutively, for example, in gastric mucosa, whereas COX-2 is undetectable in normal tissues but is highly inducible, for example, at sites of inflammation and cancer.

Although the effects of paracetamol are similar to COX inhibitors, it only has anti-pyretic properties and does not share the anti-inflammatory actions that they also possess [22]. Taking paracetamol regularly should be more effective than just taking it as required because it enables ongoing suppression of prostaglandin synthesis and thereby ongoing reduction in pain.

There is contradictory evidence about whether or not paracetamol has a synergistic effect when used with strong opioids: one study showed no benefit when paracetamol versus placebo was added to strong opioids [23]; another demonstrated a clinically important benefit in about one-third of patients [24]. It would therefore seem sensible to either continue or start paracetamol as a trial in patients receiving strong opioids. If their pain does not improve within a few days of adding in paracetamol, it should be stopped. Paracetamol comes in 500 mg tablets and the regular dose is 1 g four times a day. Continuing regular paracetamol tablets therefore requires that the patient takes eight additional tablets per day. This is a significant increase on an often already hefty pill-burden.

Adverse Effects: Paracetamol rarely causes adverse effects. The main concern is that of hepatotoxicity in overdose.

Non-steroidal Anti-inflammatory Drugs (NSAIDs)

As with paracetamol, NSAIDs work by inhibiting the enzyme cyclooxygenase (COX). However, in addition to anti-pyretic properties, they also have anti-inflammatory effects [25]. The original NSAIDs inhibited both COX-1 and COX-2, whereas some of the newer ones are more selective for COX-2 [26]. The COX-1 enzyme is produced constitutively (e.g., in gastric mucosa), whereas COX-2 is highly inducible (e.g., at sites of inflammation and cancer).

Examples of NSAIDs and Their Preferences and Selectivity
Preferential for COX-1, e.g., ketorolac
Preferential for COX-2, e.g., diclofenac
Selective for COX-2, e.g., the coxibs – celecoxib, rofecoxib
Non-selective, e.g., aspirin, ibuprofen

Adverse Effects: Although NSAIDs are very effective painkillers, they must be used with caution as they have several potentially significant adverse effects.

- *Gastro-duodenal Irritation*: NSAIDs are well recognized to cause gastro-duodenal irritation. This is predominantly due to COX-1 effects, and so selective COX-2 inhibitors were developed which had a lower incidence of this adverse effect [27]. Unfortunately, one of the coxibs (rofecoxib) led to a significantly increased rate of prothrombotic events. Other studies confirmed that this may be true of all coxibs and not just limited to rofecoxib [28, 29]. To reduce the likelihood of gastro-duodenal adverse effects, an NSAID should be chosen that has a lower risk of such adverse effects and be used in combination with a gastro-protective agent [30].

- *Bronchospasm*: Caution is needed in using NSAIDs in patients with asthma as they can provoke bronchospasm [31].
- *Renal toxicity*: Acute renal failure secondary to NSAIDs occurs in less than 1 % of patients given an NSAID per year. It is more likely if patients are dehydrated [32]. This risk is highest within the first 30 days of initiating treatment and reduces thereafter. It occurs with similar association across the different classes of NSAIDs [33].

There are many examples of NSAIDs with varying profiles and it can be difficult to know which to select for a patient. Thought must be given to the individual patient, including their likelihood of adverse effects, and then an appropriate drug chosen. Consideration must also be given to co-prescribing a proton-pump inhibitor as gastro-protection.

Opioid Analgesia

The WHO analgesic ladder divides opioids into weak and strong. This suggests that the two classes have distinct properties. The opioids share similar adverse effects and high-dose codeine is equivalent to low-dose morphine for analgesia. It may be more accurate to classify opioids along a gradient rather than separating them in this way.

Weak Opioids

Weak opioids are said to have a "ceiling effect" for analgesia, meaning that there is a dose beyond which the patient gets more adverse effects without any additional analgesic benefit. It is probably more accurate to say that as doses increase so does the likelihood of adverse effects (especially nausea and vomiting) and this outweighs any additional analgesic benefit.

When prescribing a weak opioid, the WHO analgesic ladder should be followed: a weak opioid should be added to other analgesia and not replace it (assuming it has provided some analgesic benefit). If a weak opioid is being used regularly but the patient is still experiencing some pain, then the weak opioid should be stopped and the patient moved to step 3 of the analgesic ladder and given a strong opioid instead of the weak opioid. There is no real difference in analgesic properties between the weak opioids, so if one is not providing sufficient analgesia there is no benefit in switching to an alternative weak opioid. Similarly, there is no benefit in giving a weak opioid to patients already receiving a strong opioid. Commonly used weak opioids include codeine phosphate, dihydrocodeine, and tramadol. Approximate dose conversions are shown below [34]. Tramadol is a synthetic analogue of codeine and therefore considered as a weak opioid. It also inhibits serotonin and noradrenaline (norepinephrine) re-uptake [35].

Approximate Oral Opioid Potency Ratios

Opioid	Potency ration with morphine	Dose equivalence to 10 mg morphine (mg)
Codeine	1/10	100
Dihydrocodeine	1/10	100
Tramadol	1/10	100

Conversions are approximations because of individual variation in pharmacokinetics. They should be used as a guide and the patient should always be closely assessed after performing a switch.

Strong Opioids

If a patient has tried weak opioids and their pain persists, or if they have severe pain, they should be started on a strong opioid. One common concern of prescribers, especially for patients with respiratory conditions, is that strong opioids may cause clinically significant respiratory depression. This is not the case. Pain is a respiratory stimulus, even when being treated by morphine, and it therefore antagonizes opioid-induced respiratory depression [36]. Opioids must, however, be used in an appropriate fashion – the patient should be started on a low dose (or equi-analgesic dose if already on a different opioid) and the dose of strong opioid titrated upward according to response. The body has several different subtypes of opioid receptor and different opioids work preferentially at the different receptors. However, this does not tend to guide prescribing. It should be more influenced by the patient's pre-existing medical conditions, adverse effect profile, and ease of administration for the patient.

Morphine is the first line choice of strong opioid. Sometimes it is not appropriate to use morphine (e.g., in renal impairment) in which case an alternative should be sought.

Preparations: Morphine is available in both long- and short-acting preparations. Patients should be given long-acting (modified release) morphine regularly. Most preparations are designed to last 12 h and therefore given twice a day, although some last for 24 h and are given once a day. Despite this, the patient may still experience some pain. They should also be prescribed immediate release morphine as rescue analgesia. The dose of this is calculated as 1/10–1/6 of the total daily dose or morphine. If the regular dose is increased, the rescue dose should also be increased and stay in proportion.

Starting morphine: If a patient has not previously been on a strong opioid, the dose of morphine is titrated to an appropriate level using either 4 hourly immediate release morphine (with additional rescue morphine as needed) or using modified release morphine [37]. The key points to remember are that the starting dose should be low and then titrated upward as required over a period of time and the patient should be allowed to take immediate release morphine up to hourly if required.

Titrating morphine: Morphine should start at a low dose and be steadily titrated to find the correct dose. Patients should be warned that this may take some time as everyone requires different doses to treat their pain. After starting morphine, and prior to titrating, patients should be asked if they think the morphine has provided any benefit, even if only a small benefit. If the answer is yes, it is likely that the patient has a pain which will respond to opioids and so titration is worthwhile. If the patient has experienced no benefit from morphine, even when asked to consider if there was a very small benefit, then their pain is unlikely to be opioid sensitive and alternative analgesia should be considered rather than continuing to titrate an ineffective medication. When titrating morphine (and other opioids), the dose should be increased by 33–50 % at a time. Even if the patient has required large amounts of rescue analgesia, this guidance should be followed (unless advised differently by a palliative care or pain specialist) to ensure that the patient does not suddenly receive a larger dose of modified release opioid than they require and then experience significant adverse effects [38].

Adverse effects of opioids: Morphine and other strong opioids share some common adverse effects but these are not experienced by all patients. It is prudent to warn patients of the common ones otherwise they may not expect them and then wish to discontinue the drug thinking that the adverse effects will be persistent when many of them may wear off in a few days or be preventable.

- *Nausea and vomiting*: Often occurs when starting an opioid and usually settles within a few days. As this is quite predictable, the patient should be co-prescribed or offered an anti-emetic such as haloperidol for the first week.
- *Drowsiness/lightheadedness*: Usually settles after the first few days. Patients should be warned of this and advised not to drive until these symptoms resolve.
- *Constipation*: Nearly all patients receiving opioids become constipated. This adverse effect persists. Patients should be warned of this and co-prescribed suitable laxatives.
- *Dry mouth*: Is often an ongoing adverse effect

Example
Mr H. has ongoing pain from his mesothelioma. He is on regular paracetamol and codeine phosphate. The severity of his pain was helped by the addition of ibuprofen and his pain score reduced from 8/10 to 5/10. However, the pain is still dominating his day. His pain has not changed in nature and remains a constant aching pain.

He is already on a weak opioid and an NSAID. His pain sounds visceral rather than neuropathic in nature. It would be appropriate to stop the weak opioid (codeine phosphate) and instead commence a regular strong opioid such as modified release morphine sulphate tablets.

He is on 60 mg codeine phosphate four times a day, which is 240 mg in 24 h. The appropriate starting dose of morphine would be 1/10 of this dose, in other words 24 mg in 24 h. Practically, this could be given as 10 or 15 mg modified release morphine twice daily, with an associated dose of immediate release morphine as rescue analgesia.

The rescue dose of morphine is calculated as 1/10–1/6 of the total daily dose of morphine, again rounding to sensible numbers. In Mr H's case, this would be 2.5–5 mg immediate release morphine as required.

Opioid Routes of Administration

Unless there is good reason not to, patients should be given oral morphine as the strong opioid of choice. There is no reason to give patients intravenous opioids – they are not "stronger" as is sometimes believed. They may work quicker as they do not have to be absorbed by the gut but, unless the patient is unable to absorb oral medication, oral administration should be the route of choice.

If a patient is unable to take their opioids by mouth, they can be given by an alternative route. Commonly used alternatives are subcutaneous and transdermal.

Subcutaneous

Parenteral medication is appropriate to use when a patient is not able to take their medication orally and they are not on a stable dose of opioids or rapidly require the change of route. Intravenous administration requires an intravenous cannula to be in place, which may be difficult and unreliable in some patients; patients with advanced disease often do not have the muscle bulk required to receive intra-muscular injections. The easiest and most reliable way to give parenteral opioids is usually subcutaneously.

Common indications for subcutaneous opioids include patients who are vomiting, or have persistent nausea, as they may not absorb oral medication and patients at the end of life who may no longer be able to take oral medication.

Patients requiring regular parenteral opioids should receive them via a continuous subcutaneous infusion. Rescue doses can then be given as separate subcutaneous injections.

Transdermal

Transdermal opioids are not appropriate to use in either unstable pain or when a conversion of route is required rapidly (such as at the end of life). This is because they can take at least 24 h for the patient to feel an analgesic benefit and can also take a long time to wash out of the patient's system. If someone is in the last few days of life, it is not appropriate to use an analgesia that can take 24 h to work. A subcutaneous continuous infusion should be used instead. This time-lag also makes them inappropriate to use when titrating analgesia before the stable dose requirements are known.

Opioid patches are available (fentanyl and buprenorphine) and may be appropriate when a patient is struggling with their medication (either through compliance issues or because of swallowing difficulties) and their analgesic requirements are known and stable.

Alternative opioids and when to use them

Most patients tolerate morphine and do not require an alternative opioid but there are several indications when it may be appropriate to try an alternative opioid.

Adverse effects: The main adverse effects that may require an opioid switch to attempt to resolve them are intractable constipation and neurotoxicity.

Constipation: Most patients receiving regular opioids will become constipated and should be co-prescribed laxative medication. Despite taking laxatives at high doses, some patients continue to struggle with constipation. In one study, the number of patients who were taking laxatives yet retained the same bowel movement frequency reduced significantly when patients were switched from oral morphine to transdermal fentanyl, so this is often used for such patients [39].

Neurotoxicity: Includes problems such as delirium, hallucinations, myoclonus, and even hyperalgesia and allodynia. Other causes for the neurotoxicity should be excluded and the patient should not be switched to other opioids if these adverse effects start within the first few days of starting treatment as they may settle spontaneously. If these problems persist, switching the patients to an alternative opioid such as fentanyl, oxycodone, hydromorphone, or methadone should be considered. The different opioids are chemically different and have slightly different profiles in terms of which receptors they activate. It is for this reason that switching opioid may help these symptoms. Guidance should be sought before converting a patient to an opioid which you are unfamiliar with.

Example

Mrs J. has been receiving morphine for her pain with good effect. She barely needs any breakthrough medication. She develops a viral gastroenteritis, is unable to manage her tablets, and is therefore experiencing a lot of pain.

This is likely to be a short-term problem so a solution needs to be found that is quick acting, easy to administer, and easy to reverse back to her normal medication once the vomiting resolves. A subcutaneous syringe driver containing injectable opioid would be an appropriate option as it fulfils these criteria. Commencing her on transdermal analgesia would not be an appropriate option as it can take up to 24 h to take effect and many hours to then "wash out" of her system when she is being switched back to oral morphine.

Example

Mr K's pain has been well controlled on morphine. He is admitted to hospital with a stroke. He is likely to survive, but his swallowing is likely to be impaired for several weeks, and possibly months.

This is a longer term problem than in example 1 and he may never regain the ability to swallow safely. Subcutaneous syringe drivers can be used long term but the patient may experience problems with soreness of the skin at the injection sites. It would be more appropriate to consider using transdermal analgesia, whilst considering options such as percutaneous gastrostomy feeding tubes.

Example

Miss L's pain has been well controlled on morphine. She is now in the last few days of life and struggling to swallow her medication so is worried her pain will become troublesome.

It would not be appropriate to use transdermal analgesia – her time is limited and it would not be appropriate to switch her to an analgesia that may take 24 h to work when effective alternatives are available. She should be commenced on a subcutaneous syringe driver containing injectable opioids. She is unlikely to live long enough to develop skin problems from this.

Route of Administration: Most patients are able to manage oral medication. If they are not, then it is necessary to consider if their inability to swallow is due to a short-term problem (e.g., vomiting), a longer term problem (e.g., a stroke), or because they are reaching the end of their life and now struggling to swallow. The appropriate opioid switch would be different in each situation.

Adherence: Patients who have difficulty in adhering to an analgesic regimen may benefit from transdermal opioids. Fentanyl patches are changed every 3 days and buprenorphine every 3 or 7 days depending on the formulation. They can be changed by the patient, carer, or nurse.

Renal Impairment: Most (but not all) opioids are excreted renally. If renal impairment is mild, the prescriber should be aware of this and use morphine with caution. If the patient has significant renal impairment, then morphine and codeine should be avoided, hydromorphone can be used with caution, and fentanyl and methadone appear to be safe to use. There are insufficient data about using oxycodone in renal impairment [40].

Inadequate Analgesia: May occur for one of two reasons: the patient has a pain which is not sensitive to opioids or the dose of morphine has been limited by adverse effects. It is essential to decide which of these two situations has occurred because

Alternative Opioids and Approximate Oral Potency Ratios

	Potency ratio with morphine	Dose equivalence to 10 mg morphine
Codeine	1/10	100 mg codeine
Dihydrocodeine	1/10	100 mg dihydrocodeine
Tramadol	1/10	100 mg tramadol
Oxycodone	1.5	6.7 mg oxycodone
Hydromorphone	4–5	2–2.5 mg hydromorphone
Fentanyl	100	0.1 mg (100 micrograms) fentanyl

Conversion factors are approximations because of individual variation in pharmacokinetics: they are as recommended by the Palliative Care Formulary and some differ from manufacturer's recommendation. Doses should be rounded to whole numbers.

Caution must be exercised with fentanyl doses. Confusion may arise from the numeric patch strengths. The numbers on the patch refer to the *micrograms* of fentanyl released *per hour* to the patient. For example a fentanyl "25" patch administers 25 micrograms fentanyl per hour to the patient. If a patient is receiving 10 milligrams morphine in 24 h, the approximate equivalent dose of fentanyl would be 100 micrograms *in 24 h*. If this was to be administered via a transdermal patch, 100 micrograms would need to be divided by 24 to see how much fentanyl the patient would require each hour – this would be 4 micrograms/h of fentanyl, which is significantly less than any of the fentanyl patches deliver. A transdermal patch would therefore not be a suitable option in this example. Do not make the mistake of prescribing a 100 micrograms fentanyl patch as this will deliver 100 micrograms *per hour*! Subcutaneous fentanyl may be appropriate, depending on the reason for the opioid switch. It should be thought of like any other subcutaneous opioid – the dose required in 24 h is prescribed to be administered via a subcutaneous syringe driver.

switching and increasing dose in a patient with a pain unresponsive to opioids will provide them with no benefit but continuing adverse effects. Useful questions to ask the patient include "has the morphine helped your pain at all? Even if it has not got rid of your pain, does it take the edge off it?" If the answer is yes, the pain is opioid sensitive so it is worth switching them to an alternative opioid. Approximate dose equivalences are shown below [34].

Adjuvant Analgesia

Adjuvant analgesia can be used at any point on the analgesic ladder or independently of other medication suggested by the ladder. It is often required for neuropathic pain and should be used when considered appropriate for the pain. In cancer this is usually only if pain does not respond to the combination of a strong opioid and a NSAID.

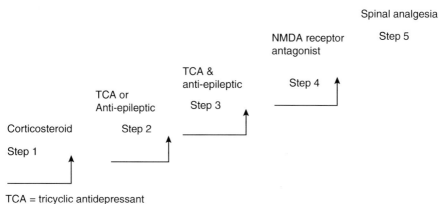

TCA = tricyclic antidepressant

Fig. 5.4 Adjuvant analgesia in neuropathic pain. These are medications that have primary indications other than pain but which also improve pain control. *TCA* tricyclic antidepressant

Adjuvant analgesics are often medications that have primary indications other than pain but work well as analgesics. For most patients neuropathic pain can be effectively managed following the WHO guidelines, including use of adjuvant analgesics. A suggested ladder for the use of adjuvant analgesia is shown below [41, 42] (Fig. 5.4).

Adjuvant analgesic drugs include the following:

- Antidepressants
- Anti-epileptics
- *N*-Methyl-D-aspartate (NMDA) receptor antagonists
- Corticosteroids
- Bisphosphonates
- Anti-spasmodics
- Skeletal muscle relaxants

There are other drugs that can be used for their analgesic effects in patients with complex pain. These are usually used by specialists, either in palliative care or persistent pain.

Antidepressants and Antiepileptics

Antidepressants and antiepileptics are often effective in the treatment of neuropathic pain but when the underlying cause of the neuropathic pain is complex, for example due to an invading cancer, it is often appropriate to try a NSAID and morphine first as in the WHO guidelines [43]. Antidepressants and antiepileptics modulate pain in different ways. If one drug provides only partial analgesia, it is worth adding in a drug from the other class.

Not all antidepressants work as effective analgesics. Tricyclic antidepressants are effective and have a number needed to treat (or NNT, that is the number of patients needed to be treated for one to benefit compared with a control) of 3.6 for achieving at least moderate pain relief. However, they are ineffective in treating HIV-related peripheral neuropathy. Venlafaxine has an NNT of 3.1 as an analgesic but a higher rate of major side effects compared to tricyclics (numbers needed to harm: amitryptyline 28 versus 16.2 with venlafaxine). There is limited evidence for analgesic benefit from SSRIs [44].

Amitriptyline is the tricyclic antidepressant most commonly used in the treatment of neuropathic pain. It works by potentiating the descending inhibitory pathways of the dorsal column. Because of its adverse effect profile it should be started at a low dose and slowly titrated. A suitable starting dose would be 10–25 mg at night, depending on the patient's frailty. This should be titrated over several weeks to 75–100 mg at night.

As with the antidepressants, different anti-epileptics have differing benefits on neuropathic pain. Although carbamazepine often works well in trigeminal neuralgia, it is less effective in other types of neuropathic pain.

Gabapentin is licensed for the treatment of neuropathic pain. It works by activating the gamma-amino-butyric acid inhibitory system. As with amitriptyline, the starting dose of gabapentin should be low and then the dose titrated upward. At daily doses of 1,200 mg or more, the number needed to treat for gabapentin is 5.8, with adverse events occurring frequently [45]. For most patients a suitable regimen would be:

Gabapentin Dosing Regime
   Day 1: gabapentin 300 mg at night
   Day 2: gabapentin 300 mg twice a day
   Day 3: gabapentin 300 mg three times a day

   Then increase by 300 mg more a day until a maximum dose of 3,600 mg/day is achieved. Many patients achieve adequate analgesia at lower doses than the maximum.
   Patients must be warned that, if at any time following a dose increase they feel unwell, they should reduce to the previous dose and slow down the titration regimen.
   In patients who are elderly or frail, gabapentin should be titrated much more slowly – in increments of 100 mg daily.

Pregabalin has been shown to be effective in a variety of neuropathic pains in doses of 300 mg/day and above. The number needed to treat is comparable with gabapentin, although varies between different conditions [46].

N-Methyl-D-aspartate (NMDA) receptor antagonists work in a way that is different to opioids, antidepressants, or antiepileptics. They are not usually considered in a patient's management until the more usual treatments have been exhausted, either through intolerable adverse effects or lack of effective analgesia. Examples of NMDA receptor antagonists are *methadone*, which also has opioid receptor agonist properties, and *ketamine*. As with many analgesics, they should be started at a low dose and slowly titrated upward according to benefit and adverse effects.

Methadone and ketamine are complex drugs that can have unusual properties. For example, methadone has a very long half-life which causes initial accumulation for the first few days before a steady state level is reached. Because they are so complex, methadone and ketamine should be started by physicians with relevant expertise, for example, palliative medicine or persistent pain specialists. Once the patient is on a stable dose, adverse effects are much less likely and the patient can be monitored by their specialist or general practitioner.

Corticosteroids help reduce the area of surrounding edema that many tumors have. Many pains that are due to cancer result from the mass compressing or invading surrounding structures, including nerves. Commencing a patient on corticosteroids reduces this edema and often provides pain relief. The benefit of corticosteroids tends to be short lived (a few weeks) and additional analgesia needs to be considered, including use of more definitive treatments such as radiotherapy. If the patient does not experience any benefit within a week, the corticosteroids should be stopped so as to prevent development of unnecessary adverse effects. Corticosteroids should not be used long-term for pain management because of their adverse effects.

Bisphosphonates are osteoclast inhibitors and may provide analgesia to patients that experience pain from bone metastases. They tend to be used when pain persists despite conventional analgesia and when oncological or orthopaedic interventions are unsuccessful or inappropriate. Benefit should be seen within a couple of weeks and patients who derive some benefit from bisphosphonates may find that this lasts for several months. Once the benefit wears off the treatment can be repeated. Benefit is more likely with intravenous bisphosphonates and in patients with breast cancer or myeloma but can be considered in other types of cancer [47].

Anti-spasmodics may help relieve distressing pain secondary to smooth muscle spasm or colic which does not respond to conventional analgesia. This may be due to constipation, bowel obstruction, bladder spasm, or other reasons. The patient will describe this as a colicky pain. As with all pains, the underlying cause should be identified and treated, if possible and appropriate. If not, then the patient may derive benefit from an anti-spasmodic such as hyoscine butylbromide. Hyoscine butylbromide is poorly absorbed orally and so should be given parenterally, usually subcutaneously in the palliative care setting [48].

Skeletal Muscle Relaxants may help relieve the pain associated with skeletal muscle spasm or cramp. On examination a "knot" of muscle can often be felt at the painful site. Non-drug treatment is best, for example, heat packs, massage and relaxation therapies, but if this pain is persistent the patient may need some analgesia. Skeletal muscle spasms do not respond to conventional analgesia, but quinine, baclofen, or a benzodiazepine is often beneficial.

Topical Analgesia

Some pains are localized, the patient may not wish to take systemic treatment or they may have had adverse effects from systemic treatment. In such patients, topical analgesia may be helpful. It is often particularly helpful in neuropathic pain. Examples of topical analgesia include TENS, lidocaine patches, capsaicin cream, NSAID gel and heat packs.

Lidocaine patches: Lidocaine is a local anesthetic that can be applied in a patch directly over the painful area. The patches are worn for 12 h and then removed for 12 h. The evidence supporting their use is not strong, but they may provide benefit for some patients. The main adverse effects are skin irritation and redness [49].

Capsaicin cream may provide some benefit in the treatment of neuropathic pain, but this is usually associated with burning or stinging of the skin. Evidence is not strong but does suggest some benefit [50].

Topical NSAIDs can be used in the treatment of musculoskeletal pain. The evidence for their use is mainly in acute pain, but shows good response with minimal systemic adverse effects [51]. This may not be the case with more chronic pains.

Heat packs can be very beneficial for patients with pain. They provide a soothing comfort, as well as reducing the pain. Care must be taken not to burn the skin.

Anaesthetic Options

Despite all the above analgesic options, some pains continue to persist and significantly affect the patient's quality of life. Advice should be sought from a palliative care or persistent pain expert, depending on diagnosis and prognosis if pain is difficult to control.

Some pains require anesthetic procedures to provide relief. These include peripheral nerve blocks, sympathetic nerve blocks, intra-thecal analgesia, or percutaneous cordotomy. If in doubt, an opinion should be sought from an anesthetic colleague who could advise on appropriateness and technical possibility of these options.

References

1. Blinderman CD, Homel P, Billings P, et al. Symptom distress and quality of life in patients with advanced chronic obstructive pulmonary disease. J Pain Symptom Manage. 2009;38(1):115–23.
2. Lohne V, Heer HC, Anderson M, et al. Qualitative study of pain of patients with chronic obstructive pulmonary disease. Heart Lung. 2010;39(3):226–34.
3. Borge CR, Wahl AK, Moum T. Association of breathlessness with multiple symptoms in chronic obstructive pulmonary disease. J Adv Nurs. 2010;66(12):2688–700.
4. Portenoy RK, Miransky J, Thaler HT, et al. Pain in ambulatory patients with lung or colon cancer. Cancer. 1992;70(6):1616–24.

5. Claessens MT, Lynn J, Zhong Z, et al. Dying with lung cancer or chronic obstructive pulmonary disease: insights from SUPPORT. J Am Geriatr Soc. 2000;48(5):146–53.
6. Deandrea S, Montanari M, Moja L, Apolone G. Prevalence of undertreatment in cancer pain. A review of published literature. Ann Oncol. 2008;19(12):1985–91.
7. Foley KM. How well is cancer pain treated? Palliat Med. 2011;25(5):398–401.
8. Grond S, Zech D, Diefenbach C, Radbruch L, Lehmann KA. Assessment of cancer pain: a prospective evaluation in 2266 cancer patients referred to a pain service. Pain. 1996;64:107–14.
9. Stute P, Soukup J, Menzel M, Sabatowski R, Grond S. Analysis and treatment of different types of neuropathic cancer pain. J Pain Symptom Manage. 2003;26(6):1123–31.
10. von der Lippe B, Sandven P, Brubakk O. Efficacy and safety of linezolid in multidrug resistant tuberculosis (MDR-TB) – a report of ten cases. J Infect. 2006;52(2):92–6.
11. Lema MJ, Foley KM, Hausheer FH. Types and epidemiology of cancer-related neuropathic pain: the intersection of cancer pain and neuropathic pain. Oncologist. 2010;15 Suppl 2:3–8.
12. Blumenthal DT, Blumenthal DT. Assessment of neuropathic pain in cancer patients. Curr Pain Headache Rep. 2009;13(4):282–7.
13. Desbiens NA, Wu AW, Broste SK, Wenger NS, Connors Jr AF, Lynn J, Yasui Y, Phillips RS, Fulkerson W. Pain and satisfaction with pain control in seriously ill hospitalized adults: findings from the SUPPORT research investigations. Crit Care Med. 1996;24(12):1953–61.
14. Brevik H, Cherny N, Collett B, et al. Cancer-related pain: a pan-European survey of prevalence, treatment and patient attitudes. Ann Oncol. 2009;20:1420–33.
15. Clayton HA, Reschak GLC, Gaynor SE, Creamer JL. A novel program to assess and manage pain. Medsurg Nurs. 2000;9(6):318–22.
16. WHO pain ladder. www.who.int/cancer/palliative/painladder/en/index.html. Accessed 30 Nov 2011.
17. McQuay H. Evidence-based medicine: what is the evidence that it has made a difference? Palliat Med. 2011;25(5):394–7.
18. Wilkinson S, Barnes K, Storey L. Massage for symptom relief in patients with cancer: systematic review. J Adv Nurs. 2008;63(5):430–9.
19. Paley CA, Johnson MI, Tashani OA, Bagnall AM. Acupuncture for cancer pain in adults. Cochrane Database Syst Rev. 2011;(1):CD007753. doi:10.1002/14651858.CD007753.pub2.
20. Robb KA, Bennett MI, Johnson MI, Simpson KJ, Oxberry SG. Transcutaneous electric nerve stimulation (TENS) for cancer pain in adults. Cochrane Database Syst Rev. 2008;(3):CD006276. doi:10.1002/14651858.CD006276.pub2.
21. Ferreira SH. Prostaglandins, aspirin-like drugs and analgesia. Nat New Biol. 1972;240(102):200–3.
22. Graham GG, Scott KF. Mechanism of action of paracetamol. Am J Ther. 2005;12(1):46–55.
23. Axelsson B, Christensen S. Is there an additive analgesic effect of paracetamol at step 3? A double-blind randomised controlled study. Palliat Med. 2003;17:724–5.
24. Stockler M, Vardy J, Pillai A, Warr D. Acetaminophen (paracetamol) improves pain and well-being in people with advanced cancer already receiving a strong opioid regimen: a randomized, double-blind, placebo-controlled cross-over trial. J Clin Oncol. 2004;22(16):3389–94.
25. Buria M, Geisslinger G. COX-dependent mechanisms involved in the antinociceptive action of NSAIDs at central and peripheral sites. Pharmacol Ther. 2005;107:139–54.
26. Turini ME, DuBois RN. Cyclooxygenase-2: a therapeutic target. Annu Rev Med. 2002;53:25–57.
27. Bombardier C, Laine L, Reicin A, et al. Comparison of upper gastrointestinal toxicity of rofecoxib and naproxen in patients with rheumatoid arthritis. N Engl J Med. 2000;343:1520–8.
28. Finckh A, Aronson MD. Cardiovascular risks of cyclooxygenase-2 inhibitors: where do we stand now? Ann Intern Med. 2005;142:212–4.
29. Topol EJ. Arthritis medicines and cardiovascular events – "house of coxibs". J Am Med Assoc. 2005;293:366–8.
30. Rostom A, Dube C, Wells GA, Tugwell P, Welch V, Jolicoeur E, McGowan J, Lanas A. Prevention of NSAID-induced gastroduodenal ulcers. Cochrane Database Syst Rev. 2002;(4):CD002296. doi:10.1002/14651858.CD002296.

31. Jenkins C, Costello J, Hodge L. Systematic review of prevalence of aspiring induced asthma and its implications for clinical practice. Br Med J. 2004;328:434.
32. Venturini C, Isakson P, Needleman P. Nonsteroidal anti-inflammatory drug-induced renal failure: a brief review of the role of cyclooxygenase isoforms. Curr Opin Nephrol Hypertens. 1998;7(1):79–82.
33. Schneider V, Lévesque L, Zhang B, Hutchinson T, Brophy JM. Association of selective and conventional nonsteroidal anti-inflammatory drugs with acute renal failure: a population based, nested case–control analysis. Am J Epidemiol. 2006;164(9):881–9.
34. Twycross R, Wilcock A, editors. PCF4 – Palliative care formulary. 4th ed. Nottingham: palliativedrugs.com; 2011. p. 355.
35. Lewis KS, Han NH. Tramadol: a new centrally acting analgesic. Am J Health Syst Pharm. 1997;54(6):643–52.
36. Borgbjerg FM, Nielsen K, Franks J. Experimental pain stimulates respiration and attenuates morphine-induced respiratory depression: a controlled study in human volunteers. Pain. 1996;64:123–8.
37. Wiffen PJ, McQuay HJ, Wiffen PJ, McQuay HJ. Oral morphine for cancer pain. Cochrane Database Syst Rev. 2007;(4):CD003868. doi:10.1002/14651858.CD003868.pub2.
38. Mercadante S. Opioid titration in cancer pain: a critical review. Eur J Pain. 2007;11(8): 823–30.
39. Radbruch L, Sabatowski R, Loick G, Kulbe C, Kasper M, Grond S, Lehmann KA. Constipation and the use of laxatives: a comparison between transdermal fentanyl and oral morphine. Palliat Med. 2000;14(2):111–9.
40. Dean M. Opioids in renal failure and dialysis patients. J Pain Symptom Manage. 2004; 28(5):497–504.
41. Grond S, Radbruch L, Meuser T, Sabatowski R, Loick G, Lehmann KA. Assessment and treatment of neuropathic cancer pain following WHO guidelines. Pain. 1999;79(1):15–20.
42. Twycross R, Wilcock A, editors. PCF4 – Palliative care formulary. 4th ed. Nottingham: palliativedrugs.com; 2011. p. 283.
43. Dellemijn P. Are opioids effective in relieving neuropathic pain? Pain. 1999;80:453–62.
44. Saarto T, Wiffen PJ. Antidepressants for neuropathic pain. Cochrane Database Syst Rev. 2007;(4):CD005454. doi:10.1002/14651858.CD005454.pub2.
45. Moore RA, Wiffen PJ, Derry S, McQuay HJ. Gabapentin for chronic neuropathic pain and fibromyalgia in adults. Cochrane Database Syst Rev. 2011;(3):CD007938. doi:10.1002/14651858. CD007938.pub2.
46. Moore RA, Straube S, Wiffen PJ, Derry S, McQuay HJ. Pregabalin for acute and chronic pain in adults. Cochrane Database Syst Rev. 2009;(3):CD007076. doi:10.1002/14651858.CD007076. pub2.
47. Mannix K, Ahmedzai SH, Anderson H, Bennett M, Lloyd-Williams M, Wilcock A. Using bisphosphonates to control the pain of bone metastases: evidence based guidelines for palliative care. Palliat Med. 2000;14:455–61.
48. Tytgat GN. Hyoscine butylbromide – a review on its parenteral use in acute abdominal spasm and as an aid in abdominal diagnostic and therapeutic procedures. Curr Med Res Opin. 2008;24(11):3159–73.
49. Khaliq W, Alam S, Puri NK. Topical lidocaine for the treatment of postherpetic neuralgia. Cochrane Database Syst Rev. 2007;(2):CD004846. doi:10.1002/14651858.CD004846.pub2.
50. Derry S, Lloyd R, Moore RA, McQuay HJ. Topical capsaicin for chronic neuropathic pain in adults. Cochrane Database Syst Rev. 2009;(4):CD007393. doi:10.1002/14651858.CD007393.pub2.
51. Massey T, Derry S, Moore RA, McQuay HJ. Topical NSAIDs for acute pain in adults. Cochrane Database Syst Rev. 2010;(6):CD007402. doi:10.1002/14651858.CD007402.pub2.

Part III
Respiratory Diseases

Chapter 6
Lung Cancer

Bernard Higgins and E. Timothy Peel

Abstract After considering the size of the problem, the chapter describes the overall approach to the new lung cancer patient in the UK, including initial treatment options. The commoner presenting symptoms are local and as the disease progresses, systemic ones such as fatigue and weight loss become more apparent. Palliative anti-cancer treatments (radiotherapy and chemotherapy) are described with particular reference to their effect on symptoms. Drug and non-drug treatment of specific respiratory symptoms are considered in earlier chapters, but there are sections in this chapter on the systemic symptoms which can occur not only in lung cancer, but also other chronic respiratory diseases. There are a number of particular lung cancer complications that need specific management strategies, including stridor, hoarseness, spinal cord compression, and superior vena caval obstruction as well as the two commoner paraneoplastic syndromes, hypercalcemia, and SIADH. The chapter finishes with care in advanced disease and carer support.

Keywords Lung cancer • Local symptoms • Fatigue • Cachexia • Sweating • Itch Radiotherapy • Chemotherapy

B. Higgins, M.B. ChB (Hons), M.D., FRCP. (⊠)
Department of Respiratory Medicine, Freeman Hospital,
Freeman Road, Newcastle upon Tyne NE7 7DN, UK
e-mail: b.g.higgins@ncl.ac.uk

E.T. Peel, M.B.B.S., B.Sc., FRCP
Department of Palliative Medicine, North Tyneside General Hospital,
Rake Lane, North Shields, Tyne and Wear NE29 8NH, UK

Marie Curie Hospice,
Newcastle upon Tyne, UK

S.J. Bourke, E.T. Peel (eds.), *Integrated Palliative Care of Respiratory Disease*,
DOI 10.1007/978-1-4471-2230-2_6, © Springer-Verlag London 2013

Introduction

More than one million people die from lung cancer every year, making it the world's leading cause of cancer death [1, 2]. There is wide variation in both the incidence and death rate of lung cancer in different countries and regions depending on socio-economic factors and the prevalence of smoking. In the United Kingdom (UK) in the period 2003–2007, there were, on average, 39,651 new cases of lung cancer registered annually [1]. Of these, approximately 42 % occurred in women, and the proportion of women affected is steadily increasing [3]. Cure rates are low, with a 5 year survival of only 7.7 % and a median survival time of only 203 days [2]. The epidemic of lung cancer is beginning to wane in the Western world but is rising inexorably in other parts of the world.

There are well-established guidelines for the investigation and management of patients with lung cancer [4]. Unless there is a specific reason not to, it is recommended that histological or cytological confirmation should be sought, the disease should be staged using the current version of the TNM classification system, and the patient's performance status should be assessed. Lung cancer is broadly divided into non-small cell carcinoma (NSCLC), the main types of which are squamous carcinoma, adenocarcinoma, and undifferentiated large cell carcinoma; and small cell carcinoma (SCLC). In NSCLC, cures are sought by either surgical excision or radical radiotherapy. Increasingly adjuvant chemotherapy is being used in an attempt to improve cure rates. In SCLC, the very few cures are achieved in patients with limited stage disease who have a complete response to chemotherapy and subsequent consolidation radiotherapy. Management of lung cancer involves a multidisciplinary approach with involvement of respiratory physicians, thoracic surgeons, medical and radiotherapy oncologists, pathologists, nurse specialists, and palliative care teams. Good communication of the diagnosis and discussion of the management options with the patient and family are crucial, and patients and their families need considerable support at the time of diagnosis and throughout the course of the disease [4].

Lung cancer management typically involves an initial phase of diagnosis during which patients and their families experience considerable emotional distress in coming to terms with a life-threatening illness. This is usually followed by a phase of specific anti-cancer treatments (surgery, chemotherapy, or radiotherapy) which can themselves give rise to significant symptoms and adverse effects. Unfortunately in the majority of cases the tumor relapses and progresses, leading to a palliative phase focused on relief of symptoms, followed by an end of-life phase. This is typical of a "cancer trajectory" and it allows a planned approach to palliative care. The importance of palliative care was emphasized by a study in the United States of America (USA) in which patients with metastatic non-small cell lung cancer were randomized to receive either standard oncologic treatment alone or with added specialist palliative care input [5]. Those receiving palliative care had better quality of life scores, less depression, and were less likely to receive aggressive care at the end of life. More surprisingly their median survival, at 11.6 months, was significantly longer than those who received oncologic care only (8.9 months). Palliative and supportive care are crucial components and must run in parallel with anti-cancer treatments throughout the course of the disease.

Presentation and Progression of Symptoms

Presentation

The commonest presentation of lung cancer is with local symptoms from the presence of the intra-thoracic tumor or from local direct spread to involve adjacent organs. Symptoms from metastatic disease are the next most common, while rarer presentations result from various paraneoplastic phenomena. Lung cancer may also be discovered coincidentally on a chest radiograph done for some other purpose. A study in 1993 reported the symptoms at presentation in 289 unselected patients with non-small cell lung cancer [6]. They are listed in Table 6.1.

While most of these reflect local disease, some, such as extrathoracic pain, suggest distant metastatic spread, and malaise and anorexia are systemic manifestations of cancer and probably paraneoplastic in origin.

Another study examined the symptoms of lung cancer patients in their last year of life and compared them with those of patients with chronic obstructive pulmonary disease (COPD) [7]. Whilst some local symptoms, such as cough, improved throughout the course of the disease, others, such as pain, became more troublesome. Systemic symptoms and low mood were common in both advanced lung cancer and COPD (Table 6.1).

	% presentation [6]	% late [7]
Cough	79	40
Breathlessness	5	69
Pain	55	64
Anorexia	45	70
Malaise	47	
Hemoptysis	35	
Hoarseness	11	
Dysphagia	7	
Vomiting		25
Constipation		42
Mouth problems		46
Insomnia		40
Confusion		33
Low mood		49

Table 6.1 Symptoms of lung cancer at presentation and later in the course of the disease [6, 7]

Mechanism of Symptoms

Cough

Stimulation of the irritant receptors in the central airways causes a cough relatively early in patients with lung cancer. The problem is that most of these people will have been smokers and possibly have a chronic cough due to co-existent COPD. The change in the nature of the cough may be an important clue. Sputum production is not discriminating except in bronchoalveolar cell carcinoma (multifocal lepidic adenocarcinoma) which is sometimes characterized by excessive secretions (bronchorrhea).

Breathlessness

Breathlessness, like cough, is a common symptom in the patient group who develop lung cancer. The commonest underlying causes are collapse of a lobe or whole lung, and pleural effusion. Less common causes include pericardial effusion, lymphangitis carcinomatosa, superior vena cava obstruction (SVCO), tumor bulk and mediastinal involvement causing a phrenic nerve palsy with diaphragmatic paralysis.

Stridor and Hoarseness

Stridor is a predominantly inspiratory wheezing sound due either to an intra-luminal tumor narrowing a large airway or from extrinsic compression of an airway by tumor mass or lymph nodes. The wheezing sound is from turbulent airflow through the narrowing. Hoarseness is usually due to left recurrent laryngeal nerve palsy from a tumor in the left upper mediastinum. This results in paralysis of the left vocal cord. In addition to a hoarse voice, such patients also develop a "bovine" cough as they are unable to completely adduct the vocal cords to generate adequate pressure for a normal cough. Rarely a tumor at the extreme right apex causes right cord palsy.

Hemoptysis

This is an alarming symptom and therefore one likely to make the patient seek medical advice. It is usually due to mucosal disruption from a central tumor or from a peripheral tumor outgrowing its blood supply and cavitating. Major hemoptysis is uncommon at presentation but can occur in advanced disease if bronchial or pulmonary vessels are invaded by tumor.

Pain

There are no pain receptors in the airways or lung parenchyma, so pain generally implies disease extension to the surrounding pleura or mediastinal structures.

Another explanation of pain is due to infection distal to an obstructing central tumor. Pleural and mediastinal pain are usually nociceptive and opioid sensitive. Unilateral facial pain due to mediastinal involvement has been described [8]. This is usually felt in or around the ear and is thought to be referred pain via the vagus nerve. It improves with palliative radiotherapy to the tumor. If a peripheral cancer invades the chest wall, it will cause nociceptive pain due to involvement of the pleura, muscle, ribs or connective tissues, and neuropathic pain in the distribution of any intercostal nerve involved. At the apex of the lung, superior sulcus cancers can either invade the brachial plexus (and cause neuropathic pain) or the subclavian sympathetic plexus. The latter is characterised by sympathetically maintained pain of the upper limb and/or an ipsilateral Horner's syndrome of ptosis, meiosis, enophthalmos and anhydrosis [9].

Metastatic Symptoms

Lung cancer can metastasize via the blood stream to almost any organ. In practice the commonest sites for symptomatic metastatic spread are the brain, bones, liver, pleura, skin, and subcutaneous tissue. The lungs and adrenals are commonly also involved but tend not to give rise to new symptoms. Bone metastases present with bone pain, pathological fracture or nerve compression symptoms such as spinal cord compression. Brain metastases can present with focal neurological symptoms due to the presence of a space occupying lesion, with an epileptic fit, with symptoms of raised intra-cranial pressure or with personality change due to frontal lobe involvement. Liver metastases are characterized by pain due to stretching of the liver capsule or jaundice if the bile ducts are compressed. Pleural involvement results in breathlessness due to effusion or pleuritic pain.

Non-metastatic Symptoms

Also known as para-neoplastic symptoms, these are thought to be caused by secretion of tumor products that act at sites separate from the tumor [10]. Some symptom complexes are not confined to lung cancer, or indeed cancer in general, but occur in a variety of advanced diseases. Fatigue, anorexia, and cachexia are the most obvious examples of this and are found in chronic lung diseases such as COPD, chronic suppurative lung diseases, and idiopathic pulmonary fibrosis (IPF). Secondly there are systemic symptoms that are more commonly associated with lung cancer and mesothelioma. These include sweats and generalized itching (without biochemical abnormality). Clubbing and its rarer companion hypertrophic pulmonary osteo-arthropathy occur in lung cancer but also in chronic lung suppuration, IPF, and cyanotic congenital heart disease. The para-neoplastic syndromes variably associated with lung cancer are listed in Table 6.2. Some, such as hypercalcemia, associated with

Table 6.2 Summary of paraneoplastic syndromes in patients with lung cancer

Neurological

Peripheral neuropathy, Lambert-Eaton syndrome, encephalopathy, myelopathy, cerebellar degeneration, psychosis, dementia

Cutaneous

Clubbing, dermatomyositis, acanthosis nigricans, pruritus, sweating, erythema multiforme, hyperpigmentation, urticaria, scleroderma

Musculoskeletal

Hypertrophic pulmonary osteo-arthropathy, polymyositis, myopathy, osteomalacia

Blood disorders

Thrombocytosis, polycythemia, hemolytic anemia, red cell aplasia, dysproteinemia, leukemoid reaction, eosinophilia, thrombocytopenic purpura, hypercoagulable states

Endocrine

Cushings, syndrome of inappropriate antidiuretic hormone (SIADH), hypercalcemia, carcinoid syndrome, hyper- and hypo-glycemia, gynecomastia, galactorrhea, growth hormone excess, calcitonin secretion, thyroid stimulating hormone

Vascular

Thrombophlebitis, arterial thrombosis, non-bacterial thrombotic endocarditis

Miscellaneous

Fatigue, anorexia/cachexia, nephrotic syndrome, hyperuricemia

squamous lung cancer, and hyponatremia, associated with small cell lung cancer, are relatively common and their management will be described. Others are much rarer and more exotic. They are more difficult to manage and may not improve even with successful treatment of the primary cancer.

Palliative Treatments

Chemotherapy

The value of chemotherapy in prolonging life in lung cancer patients was first demonstrated unequivocally in 1969 in a classic study of 2,000 patients at the Veteran's Administration Hospitals [11]. It was readily apparent even in those early days that the response rate was vastly superior in cases of small cell cancer. At that time surgery was regarded as the standard treatment of choice for all lung cancer, but in 1973 Matthews and colleagues published their experience of patients who had died within a month of surgical resection of a small cell tumor and showed that systemic metastases were present even though there had been no sign of these at preoperative evaluation [12]. In the following years it became clear that small cell tumors responded to a variety of drugs and that using these in combination produced better results than when these drugs were used as single agents alone [13]. Thus chemotherapy became established as the treatment of choice for small cell cancer.

The obvious problem with chemotherapy is the toxic effects which are both frequent and potentially serious. Even in cases of small cell cancer there has been some debate as to whether the incidence of adverse effects outweighed the survival benefit, particularly in extensive stage disease. When considering the use of chemotherapy in non small cell lung cancer, this issue becomes central. The response rate is clearly less than in small cell cancer and for years many physicians were reluctant to subject their patients to this treatment. Attitudes have changed as new drugs have emerged showing better response rates and less adverse effects. We have now reached a stage where it is appropriate to talk not just about survival benefit from chemotherapy but also about the potential benefits of chemotherapy in terms of overall quality of life.

Small Cell Lung Cancer

The concept of formally measuring quality of life was not properly appreciated when survival benefits of chemotherapy for small cell lung cancer were first being demonstrated. The toxic effects of chemotherapy were, of course, readily apparent, most notably the effects of bone marrow suppression producing anemia, neutropenia with the risk of infection, and thrombocytopenia causing bleeding or bruising. The problems of nausea, vomiting, and hair loss were notorious. Nonetheless, patients with limited stage small cell cancer who had a measurable chance of cure with chemotherapy are generally prepared to accept these, although appreciative of any attempts to mitigate the toxicity.

Reducing the Side Effects of Chemotherapy

The problem of marrow suppression is inevitable with aggressive chemotherapy, although the severity varies. The possibility of using granulocyte colony stimulating factor (G-CSF) to improve marrow function during chemotherapy has been explored [14]. In one study, 403 patients were treated with ACE (doxorubicin, cyclophosphamide and etoposide) given 3 weekly in the control group but every 2 weeks with additional G-CSF in the experimental group. Complete response and survival were improved in the intense treatment group, and quality of life was no worse. The benefit of maintaining the hemoglobin level in patients undergoing chemotherapy for small cell cancer has also been studied. Seventy-four patients with small cell cancer received combination chemotherapy with carboplatin and etoposide with or without additional darbepoetin, an erythropoiesis stimulating agent [15]. The aim in the intervention group was to maintain a hemoglobin of 12–13 g/dL. Whilst darbepoetin reduced the need for blood transfusion and improved some elements of the EORTC (European Organisation for Research and Treatment of Cancer) quality of life questionnaire, it did not produce a global improvement. Both erythropoiesis and granulocyte stimulating agents are expensive and this approach has not been subject to cost-effectiveness analysis. They are not used routinely in the UK.

Can Chemotherapy Improve Quality of Life?

Although chemotherapy agents can induce a range of adverse effects, this has to be set against their potential for shrinking or even curing the cancer, and thereby improving the symptoms produced by the malignant disease itself. Even in patients with relatively good performance status and prognosis, baseline symptoms are common. Thatcher and colleagues reported a cohort of 402 patients who were treated with standard chemotherapy regimens (ACE or carboplatin-etoposide) or with more aggressive ICE-V (ifosfamide, carboplatin, etoposide, and vincristine) [16]. At baseline about one-quarter reported their overall quality of life as poor or extremely poor. Chemotherapy produced improvements in both groups. For ICE-V the percentage with poor or extremely poor quality of life fell from 25 to 13 % at 3 months, and to 14 % at 6 months, while for the standard regime the equivalent figures were 24, 16, and 15 %. Moreover, many specific symptoms such as cough, dyspnea, and appetite improved after chemotherapy was started, although others such as general fatigue and levels of energy did not.

In a later study, Quoix measured quality of life using the functional assessment of cancer therapy-lung questionnaire (FACT-L), and also looked at individual symptoms. This was linked to a comparison of topotecan used with either cisplatin or etoposide. There was no difference in outcome between the two treatment groups, but it was noteworthy that all baseline symptoms improved with both treatment combinations, with the exception of hemoptysis [17].

The balance between prolongation of life and changes in the quality of life is perhaps most important in those patients with poor prognosis. Frustratingly there remains a paucity of good information on quality of life changes with chemotherapy in this group. A Cochrane review found only two studies of first line chemotherapy versus best supportive care in extensive stage small cell lung cancer, comprising a total of 65 patients [18]. The review concluded that the impact of chemotherapy on quality of life in poor prognosis small cell cancer is uncertain. In addition, a large study in which patients with small cell cancer of various stages were randomized to receive either paclitaxel, carboplatin, and etoposide, or vincristine, carboplatin, and etoposide, reported the results separately for the stage four patients [19]. The global quality of life parameters of the EORTC questionnaire improved. However, it is important to note that in this study patients were well enough to be randomized to receive potentially toxic systemic chemotherapy, and thus are not truly representative of the generality of patients with extensive stage disease. It remains the case that the patients with most symptoms (i.e., who have most to gain from treatment) are also those least likely to be able to tolerate chemotherapy.

Non-small Cell Cancer

The role of chemotherapy in non-small cell lung cancer has taken much longer to establish than for small cell malignancy. However, it is now accepted that in patients with a good performance status, chemotherapy confers a survival benefit. Given that the response rate is so much poorer one might have expected studies to have focused more intensely on the balance between extension and quality of life but, as with small cell cancer, formal measurement of quality of life has not been a common feature of studies until fairly recently.

Where possible, non-small cell lung cancer is treated by surgery or radical radiotherapy. There are some key questions to consider about the role of chemotherapy:

- What is the value of chemotherapy as a standalone treatment for reducing symptoms of lung cancer?
- Does chemotherapy confer any quality of life benefit if used in addition to surgery?
- Does chemotherapy confer any quality of life benefits if used in addition to radical radiotherapy?

Patients who are not suitable for surgery or radiotherapy are offered appropriate symptomatic treatment, but they may also wish to try chemotherapy rather than make no attempt to reduce the tumor burden. Among those who are fit enough for chemotherapy there is no doubt that this improves survival. Meta-analysis shows a significantly reduced hazard ratio for death, equivalent to a relative increase in survival of 23 %. In absolute terms this represents an increase in median survival from 4.5 to 6 months [20]. Although this meta-analysis included 16 randomized controlled trials with 2,714 patients, there were insufficient data to formally assess effects on quality of life. Individual controlled trials have reported either improvement or no difference in quality of life in those randomized to chemotherapy compared to those given best supportive care [21–24]. However, it is disappointing that there is no clear evidence of symptomatic benefit given the modest survival benefit.

There has been considerable interest in the use of chemotherapy combined with surgery to improve survival in NSCLC. The earliest trials which used alkylating agents tended to show an adverse affect from the addition of chemotherapy, but more modern studies have suggested that this adjuvant therapy is beneficial whether the chemotherapy is given after surgery or pre-operatively [24]. Details of which sub-groups will benefit are being refined, based on tumor stage. However, once again the benefit in terms of quality of life has not been well documented.

Chemotherapy can also be used in combination with radiotherapy as primary treatment for NSCLC. The chemotherapy can be given at the same time as the radiotherapy (concurrent chemo-radiotherapy) or one can follow the other (sequential chemo-radiotherapy). Both approaches have been studied extensively although with different drug combinations. Concurrent chemo-radiotherapy has been shown to be superior to radiotherapy alone in terms of overall survival and superior to sequential chemo-radiotherapy [25]. However, for both comparisons the concurrent chemo-radiotherapy also caused more symptoms, particularly esophagitis. Global measures of quality of life are lacking.

The assessment of the benefits of chemotherapy is further complicated by the array of drug combinations which have been used in various studies. A comparison of different regimens is beyond the scope of this book, but from the point of view of symptom palliation it is worth highlighting the tyrosine-kinase inhibitors, erlotinib and gefitinib, which act on epidermal growth factor receptors and have been shown to reduce the growth of some types of non-small cell lung cancer. They are not associated with the traditional adverse effects of systemic chemotherapy, although there is a significant instance of skin rashes which can be debilitating. They appear to represent an improvement in terms of the effects on quality of life in patients with NSCLC [26, 27].

Radiotherapy

Radiotherapy is a valuable treatment which has been in use in various forms for around 100 years. The development of linear particle accelerators began 60–70 years ago and it has become possible to link this to computed tomography (CT) imaging to deliver the radiation in three-dimensions, further enhancing the precision of therapy. This evolution continues with the advent of stereotactic radiotherapy which essentially aims to deliver radiotherapy more precisely and thus, hopefully, reduce the adverse effects which arise from normal structures being affected by the radiotherapy beam. Although important for the future, this section will concentrate on the current standard forms of radiotherapy.

Radiotherapy can be employed in a variety of ways. It can be used in an attempt to cure a lung cancer, when a high dose is employed and the patient accepts the increased risk of adverse effects that the greater dose entails. Alternatively, lower doses can be used as palliative radiotherapy with a view to reducing tumor bulk and prolonging life but accepting that cure is not likely to be achieved and that the principal value of shrinking the tumor is to improve symptoms. Sometimes there is a particular symptom which the radiotherapy is intended to resolve, and indeed this may not necessarily be in the lung, for example, bone pain due to metastasis from a lung primary is often treated with radiotherapy. Finally, there are some other specific situations in which radiotherapy has been used, for example, cranial irradiation to prevent cerebral metastases after chemotherapy for small cell lung cancer. Each of these situations will be covered in turn.

Radical Radiotherapy

Radical radiotherapy is usually given to patients who are not suitable for surgery because of comorbidity or poor respiratory function, or because they decline surgery. Dosing schedules vary, and this affects toxicity. A meta-analysis of 26 studies showed a wide variation in success rates with 5 year survival figures between 0 and

42 % [28]. As with chemotherapy, the benefits in terms of improvement of quality of life are hard to assess because of a paucity of data. One study which specifically aimed to look at this aspect of radical radiotherapy provided data from 164 patients who received 60 Gy with curative intent, and recorded quality of life using the EORTC questionnaire before treatment and then five times post-treatment up to a 12 month time point. The response rate for improvement in global quality of life was 36 % [29].

Palliative Radiotherapy

It is harder still to synthesize the symptomatic benefit from trials of palliative radiotherapy since the variation in treatment regimes is even greater, because it is not clear in some trials how bad symptoms were before treatment, because of variation in other patient characteristics, and because of variation in outcome measures [30]. One interesting UK trial looked at patients with minimal thoracic symptoms who were unsuitable for resection or radical radiotherapy. These patients were randomized to receive radiotherapy to their thoracic tumor immediately, or to wait until specific symptoms developed. Two hundred and thirty patients were randomized of whom 42 % in the delayed treatment group eventually received radiotherapy after a median wait of 125 days [31]. No difference was seen in symptoms, psychological distress, activity level or survival, implying that treatment can wait until there is at last one specific symptom needing to be addressed.

Palliation of Specific Symptoms

Cough

An unpleasant persistent cough is a common problem in advanced lung cancer particularly with more central lesions as cough receptors are present in greater density in central airways. Radiotherapy is a potential treatment option, the benefit presumably relating to shrinkage of the tumor. The success rate for significant palliation of cough is a little over 50 %, although this estimate is based on retrospective review [32]. One prospective evaluation using a standardized questionnaire found a disappointing response rate of 31 % [29]. The technique of endobronchial radiotherapy (brachytherapy) has been described in Chap. 3. It is probably inferior to external beam radiotherapy for palliation of symptoms, but has the advantage of being potentially applicable in patients who have already had maximal dose of conventional radiotherapy, the limiting factor being that the lesion has to be accessible to the bronchoscope in order to position the treatment catheters. Brachytherapy has been used to treat patients with symptomatic tumor recurrence after primary treatment with high-dose radiotherapy and a surprisingly good response rate of 77 % was seen for improvement of cough [33].

Hemoptysis

As with cough, hemoptysis secondary to lung cancer has long been treated with radiotherapy, and brachytherapy is again an option in those patients who have already received external beam therapy. Hemoptysis seems to respond well to radiotherapy. A prospective study using a validating questionnaire showed that the symptom disappeared or improved significantly in 83 % of patients [29]. In a separate retrospective study, the response to brachytherapy as second line treatment of hemoptysis was 92 % [33].

Breathlessness

Breathlessness can arise for several different reasons in lung cancer. When it is caused by the development of a pleural or pericardial effusion, or by anemia, radiotherapy has no role, nor is it of any benefit when dyspnea is caused by lymphangitis carcinomatosa. However, when breathlessness has arisen because of mechanical obstruction of a large bronchus, with or without collapse of the distal lung, radiotherapy may be of value in shrinking the tumor and relieving the obstruction. Unfortunately, even if the tumor responds, re-expansion of collapsed lung is not guaranteed. Experience suggests that expansion is less likely the longer the lung remains in its non-aerated state, and treatment of dyspnea due to obstruction of tumor should consider the role of radiotherapy in conjunction with other treatment such as stents or laser therapy. Because tumor response in this situation does not necessarily lead to lung re-expansion, the response rates for breathlessness treated by radiotherapy tend to be poorer than those for symptoms such as hemoptysis. In a prospective study, the response rate for dyspnea was 37 % [29].

Pain

Lung cancer can produce pain by local invasion of the chest wall or through distant metastases, particularly to bone. The degree of discomfort and the likelihood of a worthwhile response to radiotherapy differ a little with the extent of the invasion, but some relief is usually achieved. A response rate of 68 % has been found in a prospective study [29]. For distant bone metastases, studies have shown that a single fraction of 8 Gy is as effective as higher dose multi-fraction therapy in relieving pain [34]. Response to radiotherapy is usually reasonably quick and treatment need not be withheld because a patient is judged to be within a few weeks of death – improvement of pain at 1 month is found in 70 % of patients [35]. Treatment of bone metastases can be associated with further weakening of the bone, and this is particularly important in weight-bearing sites, such as the femur. Adequate palliation should involve orthopaedic advice, and it may be necessary for patients to avoid weight bearing for a period of time or to undergo a surgical stabilization procedure.

Cerebral Metastasis

The brain is a relatively common site of metastases for both small cell and non-small cell cancer. In the latter case, the metastasis may be solitary and in that situation treatment via surgery or stereotactic radiotherapy with a view to cure may occasionally be appropriate.

Traditionally patients with symptomatic brain metastases from lung cancer have been treated with dexamethasone with a view to reducing cerebral edema. Some physicians then proceed routinely to radiotherapy (usually whole brain radiotherapy), whereas others believe that the chances of any worthwhile benefit are confined to those who have shown a satisfactory response to dexamethasone. The evidence for this differential approach is scant. A comprehensive systematic review not confined to lung cancer found 30 trials of radiotherapy for multiple brain metastases, but many of these were concerned with different dosing schedules, the value of radiosensitizing agents, or of additional chemotherapy [36]. The central question of whether whole brain irradiation improves quality of life was not satisfactorily addressed, nor was the question of whether benefit could be predicted in individual patients. One old, small randomized control trial looked at the effects of giving patients radiotherapy plus steroids compared to steroids alone, and found no difference in improvement of performance status [37]. Survival was 14 weeks when radiotherapy was added compared to 10 weeks without, but the significance of this small improvement was unclear. A more recent study reported on the benefit of whole brain irradiation in patients with poor prognosis. This was not a controlled trial; all 91 patients had radiotherapy and completed a questionnaire before and 1 month after radiotherapy [38]. Although more patients improved (57 %) than not, the difference was modest and objective neurological status did not improve. It is therefore not clear whether patients with advanced lung cancer and cerebral metastases should receive routine radiotherapy, even though this has been standard practice. A large trial, the QUARTZ study, is currently recruiting to address this question.

Symptom Management

The management of the most common symptoms, namely cough, breathlessness, pain, and hemoptysis, are the subject of specific chapters. In this section, the commoner paraneoplastic and systemic symptoms encountered in lung cancer and, to a lesser degree, other respiratory conditions are described. The commoner systemic symptoms include anorexia, cachexia and weight loss, and fatigue. Two others, less commonly seen but equally troublesome to those affected, are sweating and pruritus. The two common paraneoplastic syndromes of lung cancer that will be considered are hypercalcemia and the syndrome of inappropriate anti-diuretic hormone (SIADH) secretion. Finally, we consider the management of the consequences of intrathoracic spread in four circumstances, namely, stridor, hoarseness, superior vena cava obstruction (SVCO), and spinal cord compression.

Anorexia, Cachexia, and Weight Loss

Anorexia (the loss of desire to eat), reduced food intake, and weight loss (of more than 10 %) are common in a number of advanced respiratory diseases. These include mesothelioma, lung cancer, COPD, and lung infections such as occur in cystic fibrosis and bronchiectasis, lung abscess, and tuberculosis. There are in fact two separate entities that result in significant weight loss in these circumstances, anorexia and subsequent starvation, and the anorexia/cachexia syndrome. The mechanisms and response to treatment vary between the two.

Anorexia and Starvation

Anorexia occurs naturally with ageing, but more so with illness. Local symptoms that predispose to it include dry or sore mouth, problems with teeth or dentures, altered or lost sense of taste, and swallowing difficulties. Other physical symptoms that reduce appetite are pain, nausea, and vomiting, early satiety due to gastric stasis and constipation or diarrhea. Depression and anxiety will also have a negative impact on the desire to eat. The result is reduced food and calorific intake followed by weight loss and ultimately starvation. Starvation is characterized by loss of fat initially with preservation of muscle. Subsequently there is protein loss, both skeletal and visceral. There is no systemic biochemical abnormality such as a rise in acute phase proteins. Management is focused on correction of the predisposing factors with appropriate nutritional support. This may be simply by improving the presentation, amount, and frequency of meals, or by nutritional supplements. These strategies should result in weight gain.

Anorexia/Cachexia Syndrome

Cancer cachexia is a syndrome defined by loss of skeletal muscle (with or without loss of fat mass) that cannot be fully reversed by conventional nutritional support [39]. In fact, cachexia is not restricted to cancer but can also be associated with other chronic respiratory diseases. The key feature is that it includes a chronic systemic inflammatory response characterized by increased synthesis of acute phase proteins and mediated by cytokines [40]. The result is redistribution of body protein with muscle wasting, hepatomegaly, and increased resting energy expenditure. Nutritional supplementation alone does not reverse the metabolic consequences of anorexia/cachexia. Nonetheless, nutritional support is clearly part of the overall management of these patients. Strategies to assist this include the following:

- Small frequent meals or snacks
- Attractive appearance, taste, and palatability of food

- Food fortification
- Oral nutritional supplementation
- Environmental issues (surroundings, social context of meals)

Various drugs have been studied in attempts to reverse the metabolic processes involved in this syndrome. Unfortunately none is entirely successful. These include the following:

- Corticosteroids
- Progestagens
- Omega-3 fatty acids
- Prokinetic drugs
- Non-steroidal anti-inflammatory drugs
- Thalidomide

It is common practice to prescribe dexamethasone (2–4 mg daily) or prednisolone (5–10 mg daily) to improve appetite (and energy) in patients with cancer-related cachexia. However, with continued use, adverse effects become prominent. Proximal muscle wasting due to the steroids is observed after only a few weeks of treatment. The potential benefit therefore needs to be balanced with potential adverse effects and survival. Megestrol acetate (40–160 mg daily) has been used with variable benefit but adverse effects include edema, feminization, and increased risk of thromboembolism.

Eicosapentanoic acid (EPA) is a long-chain polyunsaturated fatty acid in the omega-3 family which has been used in attempts to reverse cancer cachexia. A systematic review concluded that there was no clinical effect on weight, appetite, or quality of life [41]. Prokinetics such as metoclopramide and domperidone have been shown to improve the symptoms of early satiety and nausea, but do not improve appetite or weight.

Fatigue

Sometimes described as asthenia, fatigue is a very common symptom in many chronic diseases. In respiratory medicine it accompanies advanced COPD, cystic fibrosis, and other causes of chronic sepsis, lung fibrosis, and neuro-muscular disorders as well as lung cancer and mesothelioma. Fatigue includes both a physical (easy tiring and generalized weakness) and emotional component. The latter is characterized by poor concentration and memory with changes in mood. There are a number of potentially treatable causes to consider, before giving purely symptomatic management:

- Cachexia/malnutrition
- Chronic infection
- Anemia
- Chronic hypoxemia
- Emotional problems
- Insomnia
- Dehydration and electrolyte imbalance

- Other metabolic disturbance
- Drugs

In lung cancer and mesothelioma patients who do not have any of the above problems, fatigue may be presumed to be truly paraneoplastic. It is believed to be due to the production of tumor products such as cytokines.

Corticosteroids are the most widely used group of drugs for the management of fatigue in advanced disease. There is little controlled trial evidence to support their use. Dexamethasone (2–4 mg daily) and prednisolone (5–10 mg daily) are the drugs most commonly used. Certainly they have an initial positive effect, on energy and well being, as well as appetite. Unfortunately, as with their use in anorexia, the adverse effects become evident within a few weeks of treatment. The proximal muscle weakness, particularly quadriceps, then worsens the ability to walk and transfer. Steroids are therefore only recommended for fatigue for short-term use when anticipated survival is short. A Cochrane Review has examined drug treatment for cancer-related fatigue [42], Methylphenindate (10–20 mg daily) showed a small but statistically significant improvement in fatigue over placebo at the cost of some adverse effects. Hemopoetic growth factors such as erythropoietin and darbopoetin show significant benefit for fatigue in chronic renal failure only. There are concerns about the safety of these drugs and their use is not recommended for cancer-related fatigue. Neither progestational steroids such as megestrol acetate nor antidepressants such as paroxetine showed significant benefit.

Exercise programmes may be helpful for patients with fatigue. A meta-analysis of 28 studies including 2,083 cancer patients with fatigue concluded that exercise was beneficial for patients with cancer-related fatigue [43]. The nature of the exercise depends on the functional capacity of the patient and the stage of the disease, and if possible a physiotherapist should be involved as early as possible. In relatively early stages where it is hoped to restore function a programme similar to pulmonary rehabilitation may be appropriate. In more advanced disease, the aim is more supportive rather than restorative. This involves low-intensity aerobic exercise. This can be achieved with walking, static cycle, dancing, recumbent cycle or chair-based exercise. Some prefer individual activity whereas others like group work, aiming at enjoyable, purposeful, and meaningful goals. As the end of life approaches, the focus will be on conservation of energy for important activities.

Sweating

There are two types of sweat glands, apocrine, which develop at puberty and are found on the scalp, axillae, nipples, and anogenital area, and eccrine. The eccrine glands in turn are of two types, those on the palms, soles, and axillae and those over the rest of the body, which are under the control of the cholinergic postganglionic sympathetic chain [44]. It is this latter type which is involved in the excessive sweating associated with mesothelioma and other malignancies. This sweating may be due to a paraneoplastic phenomenon, in which case it will be generalized. Mechanisms for this include a response to pyrexia, the production of pyrogens by the tumor or effects of tumor products on the hypothalamus. Tumor involvement of the thoracic sympathetic chain can result in ipsilateral sweating of the trunk. Some drugs such as morphine and antidepressants can also cause excessive sweating. Symptomatic treatment of sweats includes drug and non-drug approaches. The latter includes cooling fans, tepid sponging, and wearing lightweight cotton clothes, which will absorb the sweat.

There is no drug that has been proven to consistently alleviate sweats in mesothelioma. Those which have been reported to help include the following:

- Paracetamol or aspirin as an antipyretic
- Non-steroidal anti inflammatory drugs (ibuprofen 200–400 mg 8-hourly or naproxen 250–500 mg 12-hourly)
- Propantheline 15–30 mg 8–12-hourly
- Amitriptyline 25–50 mg at night
- H2 antagonists such as cimetidine, 400 mg twice daily
- Thalidomide 100–200 mg at night

Itch

Itch, also known as pruritus, occurs in a large number of cutaneous and systemic disorders including lung cancer. Itch nerve endings are found in the superficial layers of the skin, mucous membranes and conjunctivae. Impulses pass via the spinothalamic tract, thalamus, and internal capsule to the somatosensory cortex. The sensation of itch is aggravated by anxiety, depression, and boredom, and reduced by distraction and other sensory stimuli [45]. The nerve fibers in the epidermis contain neuropeptides, such as substance P, which is a sensory transmitter. These neuropeptides also stimulate the local release of inflammatory mediators such as interleukins, prostaglandins, bradykinin, serotonin, and histamine from surrounding lymphocytes and mast cells. These mediators produce itch as well as a local inflammatory reaction [46]. The presence of a number of different potential mediators may explain why systemic drug treatment of itch is unpredictable and not always successful. Itch may occur as a paraneoplastic phenomenon, and drugs are also commonly implicated, of which opioids are probably the most relevant [47]. There is a particular distribution of pruritis associated with the use of spinal opioids.

There are two components to this, local skin care and systemic management with drugs. Achieving optimal skin hydration is important. Dry skin is commonly found in patients with advanced cancer and pruritus. Washing with soap tends to dry out the skin, so it is advisable to use an aqueous cream or add emollient to the bath water. Aqueous cream can also be applied to the skin once or twice daily. Because of the range of mediators implicated in the genesis of itch, there are a number of potential pathways that can be targeted by drug treatments. In practice, the most relevant are histamine, serotonin, and endogenous opioid. Histaminergic drugs include H1 antagonists such as chlorphenamine and promethazine, H2 antagonists such as cimetidine and mixed antagonists (doxepin). Serotonergic drugs are probably more useful in paraneoplastic pruritus [47]. Selective serotonin reuptake inhibitors (SSRI) such as paroxetine and the antidepressant mirtazapine are both effective. Ondansetron is also used in opioid-induced pruritus. The opioid antagonists naloxone and naltrexone have been successfully used for the pruritus associated with uremia and cholestasis. Anti-inflammatory and immunomodulatory drugs such as prednisolone and thalidomide are also useful in certain circumstances.

Dosing regimens:

Paroxetine 10–20 mg once daily
Mirtazapine 15–30 mg at night
Chlorphenamine 4 mg three times daily
Ondansetron 8 mg twice daily
Cimetidine 400 mg twice daily
Thalidomide 100 mg at night

Hypercalcemia

Hypercalcemia is one of the commonest paraneoplastic syndromes. In health calcium metabolism is tightly regulated by the interplay of parathormone (PTH), vitamin D, and calcitonin, their effects being mediated via alterations in absorption of calcium and phosphate from the kidney, gut and bone. This complex interplay can be disturbed in malignant disease, the commonest mechanism being production of humoral factors by the primary tumor. In the majority of cases, this is a parathyroid hormone-related protein which mimics the effect of PTH, but on occasion the tumor may produce 1,25-dihydroxy vitamin D or even true PTH. A second, less common mechanism involves direct bone osteolysis by the presence of bony metastases.

Hypercalcemia in malignancy tends to present with confusion, but sometimes with more subtle psychological problems such as depression, memory loss, or profound fatigue. This can develop into coma, made worse by dehydration which accompanies hypercalcemia. Nausea, vomiting, constipation, and abdominal pain are also frequent. The development of any of these features should prompt the measurement of a blood calcium level. The severity of symptoms correlates with the elevation of calcium level, although the relationship is fairly loose. The rate of change of the blood level is also relevant and it is worth looking over serial calcium measurements in the presence of suggestive symptoms.

Symptomatic hypercalcemia is accompanied by dehydration because the increased calcium level induces a diuresis. The reduction in circulating volume can be life-threatening, but in any case contributes to symptoms and should be reversed, initially with intravenous fluids.

The mainstay of therapy for hypercalcemia of malignancy is to give a bisphosphonate. This can be given as a single dose by infusion. Several are available; zolendronate has been shown to be superior to pamidronate which in turn has been shown to be superior to etidronate [48, 49]. Whether bisphosphonates should be used or not depends on the severity of symptoms and the level of hypercalcemia. Most physicians would certainly use a bisphosphonate if serum calcium is above 3 mmol/L, and many feel that they are appropriate at lower levels bearing in mind that bisphosphonates not only lower calcium levels acutely but also increase the average time to recurrence of hypercalcemia.

Bisphosphonates act by preventing the osteoclast-driven resorption of calcium from bone, stimulated by the PTH-like protein. There are other agents available which can help via different mechanisms, and which can be tried if the response to bisphosphonates is disappointing. Calcitonin directly reduces osteoclast activity and also promotes calcium excretion by the kidney. It is an effective calcium lowering agent but unlike bisphosphonates has to be administered continuously to be effective. Conventional wisdom is that corticosteroids do not work in hypercalcemia of malignancy, but when the mechanism is tumor production of hydroxylcholecalciferol, steroids are often effective. Furosemide can also have a calcium lowering effect by virtue of increasing renal calcium excretion.

Syndrome of Inappropriate Antidiuretic Hormone Secretion (SIADH)

SIADH occurs as a paraneoplastic phenomenon in a number of malignancies, the commonest of which is small cell lung cancer (SCLC), in which the incidence is about 6 % [50]. The clinical features of the condition depend on how low the plasma sodium level is [51]. At levels between 110 and 120 mmol/L, there are emotional changes such as fatigue or confusion, with anorexia, nausea, and vomiting. At lower sodium levels the patient may lose consciousness or have fits. SIADH may be suspected in patients with a low plasma sodium alone (less than 130 mmol/L), but it is necessary to show that the patient is euvolemic (neither dehydrated nor fluid overloaded). The diagnosis is confirmed by checking the urine and plasma osmolality at the same time. A combination of plasma osmolality less than 300 mosmol/L, paired with urine osmolality more than 300 mosmol/L, is diagnostic. Urinary sodium excretion is also raised, but it is usually not necessary to check this in the palliative care context. The other endocrine condition to be excluded is hypoadrenalism. Management of SIADH consists of the following:

- Fluid restriction (less than 1 L/24 h).
- Demeclocycline: initially 300 mg three to four times daily, reducing to twice daily. This acts by blocking the renal tubular effect of ADH [52].
- Tolvaptan 15 mg daily is an alternative treatment which acts as a vasopressin receptor antagonist.
- Treat the underlying cause.
- Symptomatic treatment of neurological symptoms.

In patients who have had SIADH at presentation of their SCLC, the plasma sodium is a good marker of disease activity. It returns to normal as the disease responds to chemotherapy, but drops again with relapse.

Stridor

Stridor is the inspiratory wheezing sound indicating significant narrowing or near obstruction of the vocal cords, trachea, or large bronchi. The obstruction may be intrinsic (by tumor) or extrinsic, from tumor or lymph nodes. Tracheal obstruction is life threatening, extremely distressing, and needs urgent management. The treatment options include external beam radiotherapy, some form of endobronchial intervention, such as stenting (Fig. 6.1), or both (very occasionally, and only in SCLC, chemotherapy may be the preferred option). If possible, endobronchial treatments should be offered, as they give quicker symptomatic relief, but the patient has to be fit enough to have the procedure. There is very little evidence comparing any of the interventions listed below in terms of efficacy), and the choice is largely determined by local availability [53].

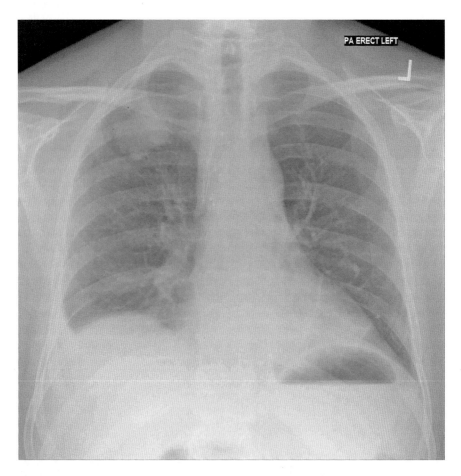

Fig. 6.1 Plain chest radiograph showing bronchial stents positioned in the right main bronchus and bronchus intermedius. The primary tumour is visible in the right upper zone and there is a small pleural effusion

- External beam radiotherapy
- Endobronchial brachytherapy
- Cryotherapy
- Thermal laser ablation
- Photodynamic therapy
- Airway stents (current standard is the self expanding metallic airway stent made from nitonol) [4]

Our experience suggests that a combination of laser and subsequent stent insertion gives prompt palliation.

Hoarseness

Hoarseness in lung cancer is due to vocal cord paralysis. The paralyzed cord is unable to adduct against the other cord and the result is a hoarse voice and the inability to close the cords prior to coughing. The resulting "bovine" cough arises because inadequate pressure is built up before the cords are relaxed. Management is by a surgical technique to fix the affected vocal cord in the adducted position. Usually this is achieved by injection of teflon® or bioplastique® [53].

Superior Vena Cava Obstruction

The superior vena cava (SVC) is a large but short vessel formed from the right and left brachio-cephalic veins. It carries the venous return from the head, neck, and arms to the right atrium. The intravascular pressure is low in the SVC and it is a relatively thin walled structure, and thus vulnerable to compression. Lung cancer is the commonest cause of the syndrome in which flow through the SVC is obstructed (SVCO) although other tumors, particularly lymphoma and thymoma, can produce the same syndrome as can rare benign conditions. Patients with SVCO often complain of cough and breathlessness, although these may equally be due to the primary tumor. More specifically, patients notice swelling of the face, neck, and arms, dizziness or headache. These symptoms may be made worse by anything which impedes venous return from the upper body, such as bending over. Symptoms are very variable, due in part to differences in the rate at which the obstruction develops. Collateral vessels may open up over time, and if the SVCO is of gradual onset, may be well established by the time complete obstruction occurs. Collateral routes include the azygos, internal mammary, and long thoracic venous systems. Dilated collateral vessels may therefore be visible on the chest wall or over the abdomen. Although SVCO is principally caused by external compression of the vena cava, sometimes clot forms in the vessel lumen. SVCO can be confirmed by a contrast CT scan of the thorax.

There is a paucity of good quality data about treatment of SVCO. Simple measures such as nursing the patient upright can help. It is common practice to give large doses of steroids, typically dexamethasone 8–16 mg/day, to patients with

SVCO. This treatment has never been formally studied and it is difficult to judge its efficacy from retrospective studies since it is usually quickly followed by some other form of treatment. Since the benefit is uncertain, it is important not to prolong steroid treatment unduly.

Radiotherapy offers a reasonable prospect of shrinking the tumor and relieving obstruction in both non-small cell and small cell tumors, and indeed in less common diagnoses such as lymphoma. When the diagnosis is known to be non-small cell carcinoma, retrospective studies have shown that radiotherapy relieves SVCO in 63 % of cases [54]. There is controversy about the use of radiotherapy to reduce tumor bulk when the diagnosis of lung cancer is strongly suspected but has not yet been proven. Radiotherapy can make interpretation of subsequent histology difficult. However, this is only an issue when SVCO is part of the presentation of a new tumor.

There are no randomized control trials comparing chemotherapy to radiotherapy for the relief of SVCO. In small cell cancers, the response rate in retrospective studies of chemotherapy suggests that SVCO is relieved in 77 % of cases [55]. The response to radiotherapy is roughly the same, and the choice will depend on whether the patient is fit enough to receive a course of chemotherapy as definitive treatment, in which case it may be best to use chemotherapy from the onset.

Self-expanding intravascular metal stents can be inserted into the SVC via the femoral or brachiocephalic veins, and offer a means of relieving SVCO even when tumors are non-responsive to chemotherapy or radiotherapy. It may not be technically possible to insert a stent depending on the presence of clot, the tightness and the length of the obstruction. However, placement can usually be achieved and case series suggest that SVCO can be relieved in over 90 % of cases [54]. Thrombolysis before stent insertion does not increase the success rate, although many centers will give Heparin.

Should stents be used in all cases, since they appear to offer the highest success rate? It should be noted that the superiority of stenting has not been tested in a controlled trial. We would suggest that stenting should be employed when symptoms are severe and rapid relief is required; or when patients are not suitable for chemotherapy or radiotherapy, including those with no diagnosis in whom rapid symptom relief is required.

Spinal Cord Compression

The incidence of spinal cord compression is uncertain but it probably occurs in <5 % of cases of lung cancer. Nonetheless, although relatively uncommon it is an extremely important condition because once established it has a devastating effect on quality of life and reduces life expectancy. Early recognition and treatment is crucial; there is a significant association between the walking ability at presentation and following treatment [55]. The commonest mechanism of cord compression is in association with collapse of one or more vertebrae. However, tumor can grow directly into the spinal cord without causing collapse, metastases can deposit directly

Fig. 6.2 MRI scan showing spinal cord compression of the upper thoracic spine due to metastatic lung cancer

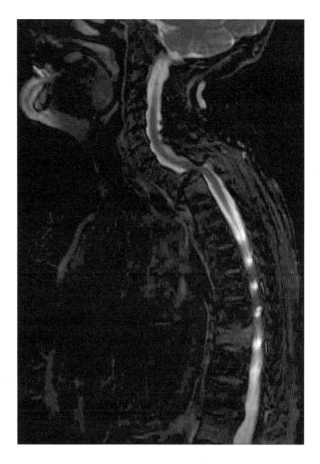

into cord structures, and in any of these situations the position can be complicated by involvement of the blood supply to the spinal cord. The rate of onset of symptoms is therefore highly variable, but the large majority of people with cord compression have reported severe central back pain for a period of time beforehand. This may be accompanied by radicular pain, and later by weakness of the lower limbs. In over half the cases, the development of sensory symptoms below the level of compression occurs. It is a sensible idea to warn patients known to have metastatic spinal cord deposits of the potential development of these symptoms so that they can report them promptly.

An x-ray of the spine may show vertebral collapse. However, magnetic resonance imaging is the optimal modality for identifying spinal metastases and for demonstrating the site and extent of cord compression. Patients should be given analgesia appropriate to their degree of pain, but urgent definitive treatment must be considered to prevent permanent neurological damage. Spinal cord decompression should probably be attempted as first choice treatment, although direct comparison with the main alternative, radiotherapy, has been mainly observational [56]. It is difficult to give firm guidance, but the choice between the two must involve an assessment of the site of the tumor and the general condition of the patient, as well as the prognosis of the primary tumor. Surgery also needs to be performed quickly as paraplegia and tetraplegia of more than 20 h duration will not recover. For most patients posterior decompression and internal fixation is the appropriate surgical procedure. If surgery is not feasible, radiotherapy may be an effective treatment, but again must be deployed swiftly. Current clinical practice in the UK is to give fractionated radiotherapy over 5–10 days, but good comparative studies of different regimens are lacking and this continues to be an area of research. When it has not been possible to give treatment soon enough to avoid paralysis, radiotherapy may still have a role as a means of controlling pain as, more rarely, might surgery in the form of spinal cord stabilization. When pain relief is the objective, several studies have shown that a single fraction of 8 Gy is as good as more complex radiotherapy regimens.

Carer Support and Progressive Disease

Patient and Family Support

Patients and their families need considerable support throughout the course of the disease. Emotional distress fluctuates, tending to peak at the time of diagnosis, when disease progression is confirmed and as the end of life approaches. Continuity of care is helpful in dealing with the different phases of the disease, and in the UK there is a particular emphasis on the role of a lung cancer nurse specialist, the primary care general practitioner, and the respiratory physician in co-coordinating care throughout the disease trajectory. In addition, a number of voluntary and charitable services are available to support families in coping with the effects of lung cancer. Many services have close links with patient/carer support groups, often run by the lung cancer nurse specialists or by bereaved carers wishing to offer experience and support. At a national level, The Roy Castle Foundation offers a variety of functions including patient and carer involvement forum, awareness volunteers, a helpline and fact sheets.

Living with Advanced Lung Cancer

Two studies have compared quality of life and service utilization in patients with lung cancer and advanced COPD [7, 57]. In general, quality of life, both physical and emotional, was maintained longer in the lung cancer patients. They had greater use of district nursing and specialist palliative care nursing services, but less social care and use of aids and appliances. The likelihood of impending death and therefore choices around this was discussed earlier and more consistently in the lung cancer patients, who were more likely to die at home or in a hospice than in hospital. In those wishing to be at home when dying, the community nurse and specialist palliative care teams are well placed to provide care and support in the patient's home.

End of Life

Compared with most chronic lung diseases with a fluctuating course, the end of life phase is more predictable in lung cancer. The recognition of this stage is considered in detail in Chap. 14. Features include profound fatigue, loss of powers of concentration or short attention span and sometimes drowsiness, confusion or agitation ("terminal agitation"). Both appetite and thirst decline, as does urine output. Of the common symptoms of lung cancer, breathlessness, cough, and pain often subside as death approaches and more troublesome ones may be agitation and noisy secretions ("death rattle"). Specific management strategies for these symptoms are considered in Chap. 14.

References

1. British Lung Foundation. Lost Lives – the UK's lung cancer epidemic. 2010.
2. Alberg AJ, Ford JG, Samet JM. Epidemiology of lung cancer: ACCP evidence-based clinical practice guidelines (2nd edition). Chest. 2007;132:29s–55.
3. Shack L, Jordan C, Thomson CS, Mak V, Moller H. Variation in incidence of breast, lung and cervical cancer and malignant melanoma of skin by socioeconomic group in England. BMC Cancer. 2008;8:271.
4. National Institute for Health and Clinical Excellence. The diagnosis and treatment of lung cancer (update of NICE clinical guideline 24) CG121. 2011. www.nice.org.uk. ISBN 978-1-84936-545-1.
5. Temel JS, Greer JA, Musikansky A, et al. Early palliative care for patients with metastatic non-small-cell lung cancer. N Engl J Med. 2010;363:733–42.
6. Muers MF, Round CE. Palliation of symptoms in non-small cell lung cancer; a study by the Yorkshire Regional Cancer Organisation Thoracic Group. Thorax. 1993;48:339–43.
7. Edmonds P, Karlsen S, Khan S, Addington-Hall JM. A comparison of the palliative care needs of patients dying from chronic respiratory disease and lung cancer. Palliat Med. 2001;15:287–95.
8. Bindoff LA, Heseltine D. Unilateral facial pain in patients with lung cancer: a referred pain via the vagus? Lancet. 1988;1:812–5.
9. Pancoast HK. Superior pulmonary sulcus tumor: tumor characterized by pain, Horner's syndrome, destruction of bone and atrophy of hand muscles. JAMA. 1932;99:1391–6.
10. Midthun DE, Jett JR. Clinical presentation of lung cancer. In: Passmore HI, editors. Lung cancer: principles and practice. Lippincott-Raven Publishers, Philadelphia, PA 19106. 1995. p. 426–38. ISBN 0-397-51361-5.
11. Green RA, Humphrey E, Close H, Patno ME. Alkylating agents in bronchogenic carcinoma. Am J Med. 1969;46:516–21.
12. Matthews MJ, Kanhouwa S, Pickren J, Robinette D. Frequency of residual and metastatic tumour in patients undergoing curative surgical resection for lung cancer. Cancer Chemother Rep. 1973;4:63–7.
13. Alberta P, Brunner KW, Mautz S, Obrecht J, Sonntag RW. Treatment of bronchogenic carcinoma with simultaneous or sequential chemotherapy, including methotrexate, cyclophosphamide, procarbazine and vincristine. Cancer. 1976;38:2208–16.
14. Thatcher N, Girling DJ, Hopwood P, Sambrook RJ, Qian W, Stephens RJ. Improving survival without reducing quality of life in small-cell lung cancer patients by increasing the dose intensity of chemotherapy with granulocyte-colony stimulating factor support: results of a British Medical Research Council Multicenter Randomized Trial. J Clin Oncol. 2000;18:395–404.

15. Nagel S, Kellner O, Engel-Riedel W, et al. Addition of darbepoetin alfa to dose-dense chemo-therapy: results from a randomized phase II trial in small-cell lung cancer patients receiving carboplatin plus etoposide. Clin Lung Cancer. 2011;12:62–9.

16. Thatcher N, Qian W, Clark PI, et al. Ifosfamide, carboplatin, and etoposide with mid-cycle vincristine versus standard chemotherapy in patients with small-cell lung cancer and good performance status: clinical and quality of life results of the British Medical Research Council multicenter randomized LU21 trial. J Clin Oncol. 2005;23:8371–9.

17. Quoix E, Breton JL, Gervais R, et al. A randomised phase II trial of the efficacy and safety of intravenous topotecan in combination with either cisplatin or etoposide in patients with untreated extensive disease small cell lung cancer. Lung Cancer. 2005;49:253–61.

18. Pelayo Alvarez M, Gallego Rubio O, Bonfill Cosp X, Agra Varela Y. Chemotherapy versus best supportive care for extensive small cell lung cancer. Cochrane Database Syst Rev. 2009;(4):CD001990. doi:10.1002/14651858.

19. Reck M, von Pawel J, Macha HN, et al. Efficient palliation in patients with small-cell lung cancer by a combination of paclitaxel, carboplatin and etoposide: quality of life and 6-years-follow-up results from a randomised phase II trial. Lung Cancer. 2006;53:67–75.

20. Non-small Cell Lung Cancer Collaborative Group. Chemotherapy and supportive care versus supportive care alone for advanced non-small cell lung cancer. Cochrane Database Syst Rev. 2010;(5):CD007309.

21. Thongprasert S, Sanguanmitra P, Juthapan W, Clinch J. Relationship between quality of life and clinical outcomes in advanced non-small cell lung cancer: best supportive care (BSC) versus BSC plus chemotherapy. Lung Cancer. 1999;24:17–24.

22. Brown J, Thorpe H, Napp V, et al. Assessment of quality of life in the supportive care setting of the big lung trial in non-small cell lung cancer. J Clin Oncol. 2005;23:7417–27.

23. Non-small Cell Lung Cancer Collaborative Group. Chemotherapy for non-small lung cancer. Cochrane Database Syst Rev. 2000;(2):CD002139.

24. Burdett S, Stewart L, Rydzewska L. Chemotherapy and surgery versus surgery alone in non-small cell lung cancer. Cochrane Database Syst Rev. 2007;(3):CD006157.

25. O'Rourke N, Roque I, Figuls M, Farre Bernado N, Macbeth F. Concurrent chemoradiotherapy in non-small cell lung cancer. Cochrane Database Syst Rev. 2010;(6):CD002140.

26. Goss G, Ferry D, Wierzbicki R, et al. Randomized phase II study of gefitinib compared with placebo in chemotherapy-naïve patients with advanced non-small cell lung cancer and poor performance status. J Clin Oncol. 2009;27:2253–60.

27. Lewis G, Peake M, Aultman R, et al. Cost-effectiveness of erlotinib versus docetaxel for second line treatment of advanced non-small cell lung cancer in the United Kingdom. J Int Med Res. 2010;38:9–21.

28. Rowell NP, Williams C. Radical radiotherapy for stage I/II non-small cell lung cancer in patients not sufficiently fit for or declining surgery (medically inoperable). Cochrane Database Syst Rev. 2001;(2):CD002935.

29. Langendijk JA, Aaronson NK, de Jong JM, et al. Prospective study on quality of life before and after radical radiotherapy in non-small cell lung cancer. J Clin Oncol. 2001;19:2123–33.

30. Lester JF, MacBeth F, Toy E, Coles B. Palliative radiotherapy regimens for non-small cell lung cancer. Cochrane Database Syst Rev. 2006;(6):CD002143.

31. Falk SJ, Girling DJ, White RJ, et al. Immediate versus delayed palliative thoracic radiotherapy in patients with unresectable locally advanced non-small cell lung cancer and minimal thoracic symptoms: randomised controlled trial. BMJ. 2002;325:465.

32. Reinfuss M, Mucha-Małecka A, Walasek T. Palliative thoracic radiotherapy in non-small cell lung cancer. An analysis of 1250 patients. Palliation of symptoms, tolerance and toxicity. Lung Cancer. 2011;71:344–9.

33. Kubaszewska M, Skowronek J, Chichel A, Kanikowski M. The use of high dose rate endobronchial brachytherapy to palliate symptomatic recurrence of previously irriadiated lung cancer. Neoplasma. 2008;55:239–45.

34. Kaasa S, Brenne E, Lund JA, et al. Prospective randomised multicenter trial on single fraction radiotherapy (8 Gy x 1) versus multiple fractions (3 Gy x 10) in the treatment of painful bone metastases. Radiother Oncol. 2006;79:278–84.

35. Dennis K, Wong K, Zhang L, et al. Palliative radiotherapy for bone metastases in the last 3 months of life: worthwhile or futile? Clin Oncol. 2011;23:709–15.
36. Tsao MN, Lloyd N, Wong R, Chow E, Rakovitch E, Laperriere N. Whole brain radiotherapy for the treatment of multiple brain metastases. Cochrane Database Syst Rev. 2006;(3): CD003869.
37. Horton J, Baxter DH, Olson KB. The management of metastases to the brain by irradiation and corticosteroids. AJR Am J Roentgenol. 1971;3:334–6.
38. Komosinska K, Kepka L, Niwinska A. Prospective evaluation of the palliative effect of whole-brain radiotherapy in patients with brain metastases and poor performance status. Acta Oncol. 2010;49:382–8.
39. Blum D, European Palliative Care Research Collaborative, et al. Evolving classification systems for cancer cachexia: ready for clinical practice? Support Care Cancer. 2010;18(3):273–9.
40. MacDonald N. Cancer cachexia and targeting chronic inflammation: a unified approach to cancer treatment and palliative/supportive care. J Support Oncol. 2007;5:157–62.
41. Mazzotta P, Jeney C. Anorexia-cachexia syndrome: a systematic review of the role of dietary polyunsaturated Fatty acids in the management of symptoms, survival, and quality of life. J Pain Symptom Manage. 2009;37:1069–77.
42. Minton O, Richardson A, Sharp M, Hotopf M, Stone P. Drug therapy for the management of cancer-related fatigue. Cochrane Database Syst Rev. 2010;(7):CD006704.doi:10.1002/14651858. CD006704.pub3.
43. Cramp F, Daniel J. Exercise for the management of cancer-related fatigue in adults. Cochrane Database Syst Rev. 2008;(2):CD006145.
44. Twycross R, Wilcock A, Stark Toller C. Sweating. In: Symptom management in advanced cancer. 4th ed. Nottingham: Palliativebooks.com; 2009. p. 331–2. ISBN 978-0-9552547-3-4.
45. Krajnik M, Zylicz Z. Understanding pruritus in systemic disease. J Pain Symptom Manage. 2001;21:151–69.
46. Pittelkow MR, Loprinzi CL. Pruritus and sweating in palliative medicine. In: Doyle D, Hanks G, Cherny N, Calman K, editors. Oxford textbook of palliative medicine. Oxford: Oxford University Press; 2005. p. 574–5. ISBN 0198566980.
47. Twycross R, Wilcock A, Stark Toller C. Skin care. In: Symptom management in advanced cancer. 4th ed. Nottingham: Palliativedrugs.com; 2009. p. 322–8. ISBN 978-0-9552547-3-4.
48. Major P, Lortholary A, Hon J, et al. Zoledronic acid is superior to pamidronate in the treatment of hypercalcemia of malignancy: a pooled analysis of two randomized, controlled clinical trials. J Clin Oncol. 2001;19:558–67.
49. Gucalp R, Ritch P, Wiernik PH, et al. Comparative study of pamidronate disodium and etidronate disodium in the treatment of cancer-related hypercalcemia. J Clin Oncol. 1992;10: 134–42.
50. van Oosterhout AGM, van der Pol M, ten Velde GPM, Twijnstra A. Neurologic disorders in 203 consecutive patients with small cell lung cancer. Cancer. 1996;77:1434–41.
51. Twycross R, Wilcock A, Stark Toller C. Biochemical syndromes. In: Symptom management in advanced cancer. 4th ed. Nottingham: Palliativedrugs.com; 2009. p. 225–7. ISBN 978-0-9552457-3-4.
52. British National Formulary bnf.org 61. March 2011:468.
53. Kraus DH, Ali MK, Ginsberg RJ, et al. Vocal cord medialisation for unilateral paralysis associated with intrathoracic malignancies. J Thorac Cardiovasc Surg. 1996;111:334–41.
54. Rowell N, Macbeth F. Steroids, radiotherapy, chemotherapy and stents for superior vena caval obstruction in carcinoma of the bronchus. Cochrane Database Syst Rev. 2001;(4):CD001316.
55. Kim RY, Spencer SA, Meredith RF, et al. Extradural spinal cord compression: analysis of factors determining functional prognosis: prospective study. Radiology. 1990;176:279–82.
56. Klimo P, Thompson CJ, Kestle JR, Schmidt MH. A meta-analysis of surgery versus conventional radiotherapy for the treatment of metastatic spinal epidural disease. Neuro Oncol. 2005;7:64–76.
57. Gore JM, Brophy CJ, Greenstone MA. How well do we care for patients with end stage chronic obstructive pulmonary disease (COPD)? A comparison of palliative care and quality of life in COPD and lung cancer. Thorax. 2000;55:1000–6.

Chapter 7
Pleural Effusions and Mesothelioma

Chris Stenton and E. Timothy Peel

Abstract Cancer is a common cause of an exudative pleural effusion. The investigation of a unilateral pleural effusion starts with simple aspiration, followed if necessary by thoracoscopy or CT guided biopsy. A recurrent symptomatic effusion can be drained, but without pleurodesis is likely to recur. If pleurodesis is unsuccessful, then an indwelling pleural catheter may be appropriate.

The chapter describes the epidemiology and presenting features of malignant pleural mesothelioma. Management strategies include preventing recurrence of the effusion, symptom control with drugs and consideration of the appropriateness of chemotherapy. There is rarely a place for surgery. As mesothelioma is ultimately fatal, there is discussion of management in advanced disease and in particular of peritoneal mesothelioma. Medico-legal aspects are also considered.

Keywords Pleural effusion • Thoracoscopy • Mesothelioma • Chemotherapy Symptoms • Compensation • Inquest

Pleural effusions are common and problematic in the palliative phase of several diseases. They frequently cause breathlessness, and they are often recurrent. They can be transudative or exudative. Transudative effusions are characterized by a protein content <30 g/L and a lactate dehydrogenase (LDH) level <200 units/L. They

C. Stenton, FRCP, FFOM (✉)
Department of Respiratory Medicine, Royal Victoria Infirmary,
Queen Victoria Road, Newcastle upon Tyne NE1 4LP, UK
e-mail: chris.stenton@nuth.nhs.uk

E.T. Peel, M.B.B.S., B.Sc., FRCP
Department of Palliative Medicine, North Tyneside General Hospital,
Rake Lane, North Shields, Tyne and Wear NE29 8NH, UK

Marie Curie Hospice,
Newcastle upon Tyne, UK

S.J. Bourke, E.T. Peel (eds.), *Integrated Palliative Care of Respiratory Disease*,
DOI 10.1007/978-1-4471-2230-2_7, © Springer-Verlag London 2013

arise from increased capillary pressure, reduced plasma oncotic pressure, or fluid overload and may complicate diseases such as cardiac failure, renal failure, hepatic cirrhosis, and hypoproteinemic states. Exudative effusions are characterized by a protein content >30 g/L and LDH >200 units/L and are caused by increased permeability due to inflammatory, infective, or malignant diseases. This chapter focuses on the symptomatic management of pleural effusions in general before addressing the specific problem of malignant mesothelioma.

Pleural Effusion

Investigation of a New Pleural Effusion

There are several comprehensive guidelines dealing with the assessment and management of pleural effusions [1–4]. A chest radiograph is the initial investigation when a pleural effusion is suspected from clinical assessment. Aspiration of pleural fluid should be considered so that the fluid can be analyzed for protein and LDH, and so that microbiology and cytology studies can be undertaken. This should be performed under ultrasound guidance to increase the likelihood of successful aspiration and reduce the risk of puncturing underlying organs. Computed tomography (CT) is the best imaging modality for assessing for pleural thickening and nodularity and for visualizing underlying disease of the lung and other organs. Further investigations may be indicated depending on the clinical circumstances.

Management of a Recurrent Symptomatic Pleural Effusion

Pleural effusions are common at presentation in patients with malignant mesothelioma. They are also frequently found in the later stages of a number of other malignancies, particularly those arising in the lung and the breast. Lymphomas, urogenital and gastrointestinal tumors are occasionally associated with pleural effusions. Persisting pleural effusions for which there is no other obvious explanation usually have a malignant etiology, and in about 10 % of cases the source of the primary tumor is never found. Intervention is commonly needed to establish a diagnosis, to relieve symptoms or to achieve permanent control by pleurodesis or the insertion of an indwelling drainage catheter.

There are risks associated with the manipulation of pleural effusions such as causing damage to underlying organs or introducing infection into the pleural space. Pleural procedures should only be carried out by those with adequate training and experience, and with ultrasound guidance. Phrenic nerve paralysis, pleural fibrosis, and lung problems can all mimic pleural effusions on a chest radiograph and several studies have demonstrated that clinicians are poor at determining the optimum or even an appropriate site to insert a chest drain or needle for aspiration. Unless infection is suspected, aspirating a pleural effusion is rarely an emergency and it should generally be carried out as a planned procedure during normal working hours when support is likely to be available. Aseptic technique is important and there is a risk of significant bleeding unless clotting abnormalities are corrected and the effect of anticoagulants reversed. Written informed consent should generally be obtained from the patient before any invasive pleural procedure.

Larger Volume Pleural Aspirate: For Symptomatic Relief

Larger volumes of pleural fluid can be removed to relieve breathlessness using a plastic intravenous cannula connected via a three-way tap to a syringe and a collecting bag. There are also commercially available pleural aspiration sets containing the necessary equipment. The larger size of the needle and the longer duration of the procedure compared with a small volume diagnostic aspirate necessitate the use of local anesthetic. One percent lidocaine should be used, taking care to infiltrate deeply to just below the parietal pleura. It is important that patients are comfortable as they are likely to have to maintain their posture for 10–20 min. If sitting forward they should have a table or chair to lean on and should be able to flex their knees. Explanation and reassurance may be needed throughout the procedure. Aspiration of fluid often needs to be carried out more posteriorly than the triangle of safety used with pneumothoraces but it is important not to aspirate too medially as the intercostal vessels frequently loop below the lower margin of their rib posteriorly [1].

Faintness or nausea caused by vasovagal reactions are common but are usually short-lived. Generally pleural aspiration becomes uncomfortable and causes coughing after about a liter of fluid has been removed. Severe coughing is an indication to stop the procedure. No more than 1.5 L should be removed at any time because of the risk of provoking re-expansion pulmonary oedema which can be severe and on rare occasions fatal.

Pleural fluid generally re-accumulates after aspiration and the relief of breathlessness is often short-lived. Repeated aspiration can be used in those who are frail and have a limited life expectancy, and often fluid reaccumulation becomes less troublesome as a tumor progresses and obliterates the pleural cavity. In general, however, a chemical pleurodesis or the insertion of an indwelling catheter is preferable to repeated aspiration.

Intercostal Chest Drainage and Pleurodesis

Small bore rather than large bore chest drains should be used as they are just as effective and cause less discomfort [1]. The pleural effusion should be drained to dryness, removing no more than 1.5 L at any time. Sometimes the lung fails to re-expand because of overlying tumor ("trapped lung") and the pleural cavity fills with air (Fig. 7.1). Pleurodesis will not be effective under those circumstances as the visceral and parietal pleural cannot be opposed. A variety of sclerosing agents can

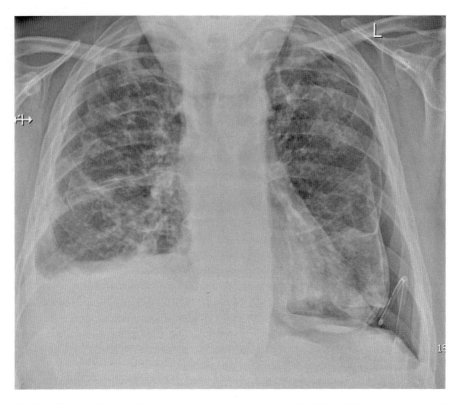

Fig. 7.1 Chest radiograph showing a trapped and partly deflated left lung following aspiration of pleural fluid with a small bore chest drain. Small right-sided pleural effusion

be used for pleurodesis but sterile talc (3–5 g made up as a slurry in 50 mL saline) is the most effective. Sclerosing agents can provoke severe pain and their use should be preceded by the intrapleural instillation of lidocaine. Premedication with sedatives and analgesics should also be considered. Systemic corticosteroids and possibly non-steroidal anti-inflammatory drugs reduce the effectiveness of sclerosing agents. Their use is not a contraindication to pleurodesis but if possible they should be stopped prior to the procedure. A range of effectiveness has been reported for talc pleurodesis but an 80 % success rate should be achievable with proper attention to technique.

Video-Assisted Pleural Biopsy and Pleurodesis

Video-assisted thoracoscopy can be carried out under either local anesthesia with sedation or under general anesthesia. It can combine a pleural biopsy, drainage of an effusion and pleurodesis in one procedure. It is not without significant morbidity. It typically requires chest drainage for 3–7 days and a total hospital stay of 7–8 days.

About 15 % of patients experience complications such as persisting air leakage, persisting pain, or less commonly pleural infection or pneumonitis [5]. The patient's overall state of health and the likely benefits need to be considered prior to the procedure.

Indwelling Catheters

Tunneled indwelling pleural catheters are a useful option in those with "trapped lung," or failed chemical pleurodesis. The catheter can be placed as a day case procedure rather than requiring an inpatient stay in hospital, and this can be of considerable benefit to those with a limited life expectancy. The catheter can be connected to a collecting bottle which is drained as necessary [1]. Complete control of breathlessness is reported in two-thirds of patients. Complications such as loculation of the pleural fluid occur in about 18 % of patients, and infection in about 6 %. Occasionally tumor will seed along the catheter track.

Malignant Mesothelioma

Malignant mesothelioma is a primary tumor of the pleura and occasionally of the peritoneum or pericardium. It is rapidly progressive, surgically incurable, and poorly responsive to radiotherapy and chemotherapy. It affects an increasingly aged population who often have substantial comorbidities. Palliative care is an important consideration for all patients from the time their tumor presents. Pain and breathlessness are the usual presenting symptoms and sweating is often a prominent feature. Psychological and emotional problems are common at the time of diagnosis and as the disease progresses, and patients and their families require substantial support throughout the course of the disease. There are often legal and compensation issues to contend with on account of the tumor's close association with previous occupational asbestos exposures.

Epidemiology and Pathology

Mesotheliomas are closely associated with work with asbestos and are around 1,000 times more common in those with typical occupational exposures. Asbestos was widely used in transport, construction, and industry in the second half of the twentieth century on account of its structural and insulating properties. The current worldwide mesothelioma epidemic reflects exposures from those sources. Mesotheliomas can occur after radiotherapy and occasionally appear to arise spontaneously but many if not all of these are caused by environmental asbestos exposure.

The risk of mesothelioma increases with the extent of previous asbestos exposure but this is often difficult to quantify accurately and the relationship appears relatively weak. The tumor can occur following low-level exposures, for example, from washing the clothing of a family member. Crocidolite (blue) and amosite (brown) asbestos persist longer in the lung and are considerably more potent causes of mesothelioma than white (chrysotile) asbestos. The relatively low risk associated with the latter may be entirely due to its contamination with another asbestos fiber, tremolite. Industrial workers generally had mixed exposures and the epidemiology of mesothelioma is dominated by the time from first exposure. The risk increases exponentially with time and so mesotheliomas are rare within 20 years of first exposure and occur on average after about 40 years. Most patients are over 70 years of age at presentation. Men are affected five times as often as women reflecting their greater occupational exposures.

Because asbestos exposures came under increasingly stringent control from the early 1970s onwards mesothelioma incidence is currently around its peak in most industrialized countries. In the UK, there are approximately 2,500 cases per annum. The UK rate is five times higher than that in the USA and the total numbers of cases are similar in the two countries despite their different populations. The rates in other European countries are also lower than in the UK, the latter's high rate being attributed to its greater and more prolonged use of amosite asbestos. Incidences in younger age groups have fallen most in recent years, reflecting better control of their asbestos exposures. As incidence falls, so the average age of those with mesotheliomas will increase and by 2030 most patients are likely to be more than 80 years old. This will influence the approach to the management of the tumor.

Histologically, mesotheliomas can have an epitheliod, sarcomatoid, or a mixed appearance with epithelioid tumors having a better prognosis. Usually they can be differentiated from metastatic pleural carcinomas by their light microscopic appearances and immunohistochemical staining pattern but poorly differentiated tumors are sometimes difficult to characterize. Differentiation from benign reactive pleuritis or pleural fibrosis can be difficult and approximately 10 % of pleural biopsies that show benign features only are falsely negative and subsequently turn out to be malignant [6].

Mesotheliomas usually present with large pleural effusions that cause breathlessness and sometimes chest pain. Occasionally there is solid pleural tumor only. They generally spread diffusely throughout the pleural cavity leading to encasement of the lung. Direct spread to adjacent organs and through the chest wall is common, particularly along the tracks of biopsies and through incisions. Distant metastases are frequently found at autopsy but they rarely give rise to symptoms. Progression is usually rapid with median survival in the region of 12 months for epithelioid and 6 months for sarcomatoid tumors [7]. A recent study from Australia confirmed the survival difference between epithelioid and sarcomatoid tumors [8]. It also showed that those with peritoneal mesothelioma had a worse median survival, at 16 weeks, than pleural (36 weeks). Finally, it reported an improvement in survival by decade from 25 weeks in 1970–1979 to 43 weeks from 2000 to 2005. This may be due to diagnosis of the tumor at an earlier stage. A few patients survive for several years and untreated survival of up to 10 years has been reported.

Presentation and Symptoms

Given its doubling time, most mesotheliomas are likely to have been present subclinically for 10 years or so by the time of diagnosis. Occasionally the tumor is identified on a radiograph or CT scan obtained for some other purpose but for most individuals it is the abrupt onset of breathlessness associated with a pleural effusion and chest pain that brings the tumor to light. Abdominal symptoms predominate in peritoneal mesotheliomas.

The presenting symptoms in patients with pleural mesothelioma, are mostly physical. Because of the subsequent realization of its association with previous occupation and the poor prognosis, emotional issues become more prominent with the progression of the disease. These affect both patient and carer.

Presenting Symptoms

In early disease, local symptoms predominate over systemic ones. Of these, pain and breathlessness are the commonest, but cough is also described. The prevalence of these symptoms varies in different series [9]. Pain has been reported in 29–85 %, breathlessness in 28–89 %, and both in 89–96 % of patients at presentation. Cough is reported in 16–75 %. The most prominent systemic symptoms are fatigue, anorexia, weight loss, and sweating. These tend to become more prominent as the disease progresses.

The pain of mesothelioma can be nociceptive, neuropathic, or sympathetically maintained. As the tumor usually originates in the parietal pleura, localized opioid sensitive pain is common, particularly if there is no associated pleural effusion. As it progresses, the tumor invades surrounding structures. Outwardly this involves the chest wall with compression or destruction of the intercostal nerves, resulting in neuropathic pain, as well as muscle, ribs, subcutaneous tissues, and skin. Medially the mediastinal structures and vertebral column can be affected. At the thoracic inlet, involvement of the brachial plexus results in neuropathic pain, and involvement of the subclavian sympathetic chain causes sympathetically maintained pain of the arm.

Breathlessness is usually initially due the presence of a pleural effusion, and responds to removal of that fluid. With disease progression the pleural tumor encases and restricts expansion of the affected lung. When this happens, more general dyspnea-management strategies are needed. Mesothelioma can also affect the pericardium, causing pericardial effusion or tamponade. This can be managed acutely by pericardial aspiration or for the longer term by the formation of a pericardial window. A less common cause of breathlessness is phrenic nerve damage, due to mediastinal invasion, resulting in diaphragmatic paralysis.

Cough is due to pleural irritation, and is usually dry. It is commonly encountered towards the end of pleural aspiration and is often the indicator to halt the procedure. Opioids are the drug treatment of choice for this type of troublesome cough.

Although mesothelioma can and does metastasize via the bloodstream, symptoms of distant spread rarely predominate over local ones. A more likely complication of advancing disease is of penetration of the tumor through the diaphragm with ascites and intra-abdominal lymphadenopathy.

Systemic Symptoms

Emotional symptoms are common. These include anxiety, fear, anger, and depression. The prevalence of these has been reported at between 20 and 67 % in patients and 57 to 84 % of carers [10]. Anorexia and weight loss are less common at presentation, but tend to become more prevalent as the disease progresses. Prevalence has been reported at between 3 and 87 %. The symptoms are probably a manifestation of the anorexia/cachexia syndrome rather than starvation due to loss of appetite with subsequent low calorific intake alone.

Fatigue is another symptom which tends to become more prominent with progressive disease. It has been reported in 32–94 % of patients. Fever and sweats seem to be more prevalent in mesothelioma patients than in those with lung cancer. Fever has been reported in 3–9 % patients at diagnosis and sweats in 20 %. Again the symptoms worsen with advancing disease. Details of the management of these symptoms are given in Chap. 6.

Approach to the Patient with Suspected Mesothelioma

The management of malignant mesotheliomas is primarily palliative. They are rapidly progressive, are almost universally fatal, and have no treatment that markedly prolongs life. The typical patient is elderly and has comorbidities. Fewer than 50 % of patients have World Health Organization performance status of 0 or 1 at presentation, indicating that they are unable to carry out the equivalent of light housework [7]. A quarter have comorbidities sufficiently severe to preclude any form of active treatment. An early balance may have to be struck between undertaking invasive investigations and living with diagnostic uncertainty, between symptom control and attempts at modifying the course of the disease, and between maintaining a positive approach and tempering unrealistic expectations.

The diagnosis of mesothelioma may be strongly suspected if someone with a history of asbestos exposure or asbestos pleural plaques on a chest radiograph presents with a unilateral pleural effusion, particularly if that is associated with chest pain and some weight loss. The history of asbestos exposure may need to be actively sought as many patients initially deny exposure and only recall it later after detailed enquiry. The relevant exposures may have been brief, may have occurred indirectly from other workers using asbestos in the vicinity or even from domestic contact, and may have occurred more than half a century earlier. The risk of developing a malignant mesothelioma is in the region of 2 % for most asbestos-exposed workers though historically some groups who were heavily exposed to crocidolite asbestos had much higher rates than that.

Even if the diagnosis of mesothelioma is strongly suspected, alternatives such as cardiac failure, tuberculosis, or rheumatoid pleural disease need to be considered as their management is very different from that of suspected pleural malignancy. More often the principal differential diagnoses will be of a benign asbestos-induced pleural effusion or a secondary pleural adenocarcinoma. A number of very rare primary pleural sarcomas are described.

Asbestos can cause benign pleural effusions that resolve, leaving diffuse pleural fibrosis. The risk for typical asbestos-exposed workers is around 2 %, which is similar to their risk of developing a mesothelioma. Benign asbestos-induced pleural effusions can be asymptomatic but they are often associated with breathlessness. They can be clinically very difficult to distinguish from mesotheliomas, though they are less likely to be associated with chest pain or systemic malaise. They frequently present sequentially, affecting one side and then after an interval of several months the contralateral side. That helps clarify the diagnosis as mesotheliomas are almost never bilateral. There is no effective treatment.

The pleural cavity is a common site for metastases from lung and breast tumors, and occasionally from stomach, kidney, ovary, and prostate cancers. Metastatic pleural adenocarcinomas often present with pleural effusions and appear clinically and radiologically similar to mesotheliomas. The pleural involvement renders the primary tumor surgically incurable though it may still be amenable to chemotherapy. Thus, even if the pleural disease appears clearly malignant, obtaining a histological diagnosis may help guide treatment.

Diagnostic Investigations

A chest radiograph will almost always be obtained from a patient presenting with a suspected pleural malignancy. A diagnostic pleural aspirate can be easily obtained in the out-patient clinic but the test is relatively insensitive, identifying malignant cells in only 30–50 % of mesotheliomas [11]. Computed tomography (CT) is associated with little additional morbidity and should generally be considered. Features such as nodularity of the pleural shadowing or extension of pleural shadowing onto the mediastinal surface suggest malignancy rather than benign disease though they do not differentiate mesotheliomas from metastatic pleural tumors (Fig. 7.2). If there is an identifiable pleural mass, it can be biopsied under CT guidance and this will identify around 80–85 % of mesotheliomas. If breathlessness is a significant problem and the patient's general physical condition allows it, then a thoracoscopy with pleural aspiration, biopsy, and pleurodesis is likely to be the most rapid way of achieving a diagnosis and symptom control.

A frank discussion will generally be necessary around this stage. Given the limited effectiveness of the current therapeutic options, some patients will prefer uncertainty and limited intervention while others will want to be as certain as possible of the diagnosis

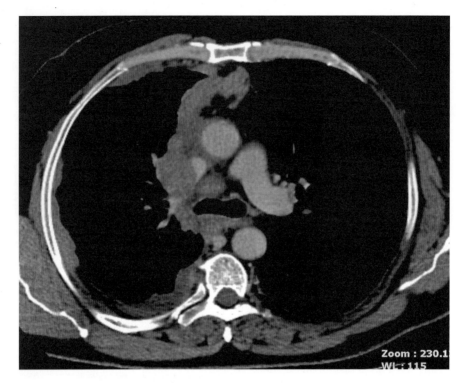

Fig. 7.2 CT scan at mid thoracic level of right-sided malignant mesothelioma with irregular pleural shadowing particularly involving the mediastinal surfaces. Some reduction of the right lung volume

and will seek every possibility of slowing the progression of the tumor. They should be allowed sufficient time to understand the information and offered the support of a multidisciplinary team. If the histology of the tumor is known, that will help inform the patient about the likely prognosis. General wellbeing (performance status) at presentation and the presence of hematological abnormalities are also related to survival [12].

Chemotherapy

The commonest treatment decision is whether or not to consider chemotherapy. It is generally accepted that only patients with a WHO performance status of 0–1 are suitable for this.

There is only one large placebo controlled study of chemotherapy as primary treatment for mesothelioma [13]. It showed a small and non-significant survival benefit (8.5 versus 7.6 months) but that was with a treatment regimen (Mitomycin, Vinblastine and Cisplatin) that would now be considered suboptimal. There were improvements in patients' pain and sweating but these were offset by higher levels of lethargy, alopecia, and hematological complications, and there were no substantial differences in quality of life measures. Raltitrexed with cisplatin increased survival by 2 months compared with cisplatin alone in another randomized study [14]. There was better relief of symptoms by the more active treatment, though the effect on patients' overall quality of life was uncertain. Treatment with cisplatin and pemetrexed resulted in a median survival of 12.1 months compared with 9.3 months in those treated with cisplatin alone in a third study [15]. Hematological and gastrointestinal side-effects were common but could be reduced by vitamin supplementation. Cisplatin/pemetrexed is now the most widely used regimen in the UK.

About one-third of mesothelioma patients are sufficiently fit at presentation to receive chemotherapy and they should be offered treatment [7]. When advising patients it seems reasonable to suggest that chemotherapy on average prolongs life in the region of 3–4 months and improves symptoms at the expense of the inconvenience and side-effects of the chemotherapy itself. There is likely to be a range of responses with some patients doing better than average and others worse. The extent of that range is not known and there are no features that can be used to predict an individual's response. Only about half of patients who were considered fit for chemotherapy elected to have it in one study [13].

Some patients are reluctant to start chemotherapy at an early stage in their illness when they are relatively well, and wish to defer treatment until they become more symptomatic. It is not known whether the response is better when given early. There is one small study that suggests a non-significant improvement of 3 months in the time to symptom progression, and a 4 month improvement in survival in those randomized to early treatment, but there were no differences in quality of life measures [16]. Patients' clinical condition can deteriorate rapidly and deferring chemotherapy runs a risk of them never receiving it.

Radiotherapy

Mesotheliomas are relatively radio-resistant and there is no role for radical radiotherapy in the treatment of intrathoracic disease. Localized radiotherapy can be used to treat chest wall pain or tumors growing through the chest wall. It is effective in about 50 % of patients, though the effects are often short-lived. Because of the tendency of mesothelioma to grow along biopsy tracts, prophylactic radiotherapy is sometimes given though there are differences in opinion about its effectiveness [17, 18].

A Cochrane review identified no randomized controlled trials showing that radiotherapy is an effective option for pleural mesothelioma [19].

Surgery

Two surgical approaches have been used in attempts to cure mesotheliomas: extrapleural pneumonectomy and pleurectomy with decortication. Information about them is readily available and informed patients often consider the possibility of a surgical cure. Extrapleural pneumonectomy involves resection of the lung, pleura, hemi-diaphragm, and the pericardium. It is technically challenging and is associated with up to 10 % perioperative mortality and significant complications in around 50 % of patients [20]. Pleurectomy with decortication involves the removal of all gross disease from the pleural surfaces but preservation of the underlying lung. Surgery is generally combined with chemotherapy and/or radiotherapy in "multimodality treatment." Occasional "cures" and prolonged survivals are reported but those undergoing surgery are highly selected and generally have a number of favorable prognostic features in any case. There is no evidence of any overall survival benefit [21]. Some younger fitter patients will want to try radical treatment, and that may be important in maintaining their morale. For most, the search for a cure will be illusory and may distract from symptom relief.

Psychological and Legal Aspects

A diagnosis of malignancy is associated with a variety of emotional and psychological responses including fear, guilt, anger, and depression. The response to mesothelioma can differ or be exaggerated for a number of reasons. Unlike lung cancer and other malignancies, the patient generally bears no responsibility for their tumor and thus can escape the guilt that is associated, for example, with previous smoking. Anger at the employer whose exposures cause the mesothelioma might be expected but is relatively uncommon and patients' attitudes generally remain neutral or include gratitude at having been provided with a steady source of income [9]. Mesotheliomas cluster in specific occupational groups and at diagnosis patients often have had experience of others with the tumor. This can heighten anxiety about their own clinical course. Mesotheliomas generally have a reputation as a particularly unpleasant illness and some patients may have anxieties about occupational asbestos exposures long before their tumor develops.

Moore and colleagues quantified emotional functioning in patients with mesotheliomas and their families [9]. They recorded anxiety in two-thirds of patients and depression, fear, and isolation in about half. Carers had higher levels of emotional morbidity with about 80 % reporting anxiety and depression. Most patients (71 %) ultimately felt peace or acceptance but only a minority of carers (23 %) did so. Thus, particularly in the early stage of the disease, attention should be paid to the patient's need for psychological support. Patient support groups can play an important supportive role and information about them should be made available.

Because most mesotheliomas are caused by work there are systems for compensating sufferers in most countries. These can form part of the state benefits system or involve civil litigation. Patients are likely to need professional legal guidance to assist them with a number of complex issues.

In the UK, state compensation for malignant mesothelioma is available principally through the Industrial Injury Benefits scheme. Benefit is paid at approximately 150 % of the state pension level for the remainder of life. The benefit applies to employees and there is a separate scheme for those who were exposed whilst in the armed forces. A lump sum can be paid to those who were self-employed or who are unable to obtain compensation in the civil courts because the employer or his insurer cannot be identified, or is no longer in business. Mesothelioma patients remain entitled to additional benefits available to those who require support because of disability, cancer, or other advanced illnesses. Industrial Injury Benefit is not means tested but an award can affect the value of other means tested benefits.

Awards made by civil courts for damages from an employer or insurer can be more substantial than those of the state scheme when, for example, they take into account loss of earnings caused by premature death. Claims have been challenged by insurers on a number of complex legal issues relating to responsibility for the mesothelioma: What extent of exposure is needed to consider an employer responsible? Is it the insurer at the time of exposure, or at the time the tumor develops, who is responsible? If there is more than one employer how is responsibility shared? Patients should seek advice from an experienced attourney to assist with these and other matters.

Care in Advanced Disease

Physical Symptoms in Pleural Mesothelioma

The only disease-modifying treatment that patients with mesothelioma are likely to receive is chemotherapy, if fit enough. When the disease progresses they may be offered further treatment if their performance status is adequate, but inevitably there will come a time when symptom management and social care become the priority. As mentioned previously, the commoner physical symptoms in advanced mesothelioma are as follows:

- Breathlessness (Chap. 2)
- Pain (Chap. 5)
- Fatigue (Chap. 6)
- Anorexia and cachexia (Chap. 6)
- Sweats (Chap. 6)
- Cough (Chap. 4)

Percutaneous Cervical Cordotomy

The pain of mesothelioma can be complex and very troublesome. It is often a combination of nociceptive pain from pleural and chest wall invasion and neuropathic pain from infiltration of the intercostal nerves, brachial plexus, or even spinal cord. Sometimes good pain control is not achieved, even with a combination of opioids and drugs for neuropathic pain, because of lack of adequate effect or unacceptable adverse effects. In these circumstances, neurolytic blockade may be appropriate. One such technique is percutaneous cervical cordotomy. In this procedure, the contralateral anterolateral spinothalamic tract is interrupted at the C1/2 level by thermocoagulation. The procedure has a good success rate with 38 % of patients being able to stop their opioids and is safe with no treatment related deaths or major complications reported in one study [22]. Sadly there are currently only four centers in the UK providing this service [23].

Management of Peritoneal Mesothelioma

Peritoneal mesothelioma usually presents with abdominal pain and ascites. As it progresses there are increasing problems with bowel transit due to the presence of peritoneal tumor. Subacute and ultimately complete bowel obstruction may occur as terminal events.

Management of Malignant Ascites

In principle, management options for malignant ascites include paracentesis, diuretics, peritoneovenous shunts, and tunneled indwelling peritoneal catheters. A systematic review of these options examined 32 studies of 849 patients [24]. Paracentesis was shown to give good but temporary relief in up to 90 % of patients. There was no consensus about speed of fluid withdrawal, and intravenous fluid replacement was not usually necessary if less than 5 L was being removed unless the patient was hypotensive or dehydrated. There is no clear role for intravenous albumin either. Shunt insertion is associated with potentially serious adverse effects and is only recommended when other options have failed [24].

Diuretics are often given with the aim of slowing reaccumulation of the fluid. A survey of clinical practice showed that 98 % of clinicians used paracentesis and 61 % diuretics [25]. The most commonly used diuretics were furosemide and spironolactone, with spironolactone being the preferred. Doses were not specified but in practice doses of spironolactone of up to 200 mg are sometimes used. The evidence supporting any of the interventions used in managing malignant ascites is weak, largely because of the poor quality of the evidence base [24].

Impending Bowel Obstruction

Because of the risk of bowel obstruction, it is important to give adequate laxatives to maintain stool consistency on the loose side. Docusate (a softener and stimulant laxative) is commonly used initially. Osmotic laxatives such as polyethylene glycol are also appropriate. The dose cannot be predicted for an individual patient and dose titration is necessary. To improve bowel transit it is often appropriate to add a prokinetic agent such as metoclopramide or domperidone orally.

As the disease progresses, symptoms of subacute obstruction such as abdominal colic, increased distension, noisy bowel sounds, vomiting, and constipation may appear. These can be managed by converting the prokinetic drug to a continuous subcutaneous infusion (CSCI) of metoclopramide (30 mg/24 h, titrated up to a maximum of 120 mg/24 h), with high-dose subcutaneous dexamethasone (8 mg twice daily) and additional laxatives.

Ultimately the patient may well obstruct completely. Here the focus of management shifts to purely symptom control. Colic may be palliated by a CSCI of hyoscine butyl bromide starting at 60 mg/24 h, titrated up to 120 mg/24 h if necessary. Intestinal secretions can be reduced by a CSCI of octreotide 300 micrograms/24 h, titrated upward; the antiemetic of choice is cyclizine CSCI 150 mg/24 h. Any other drugs needed, such as analgesics, should also be given by CSCI. Feculent vomiting is a distressing symptom and cannot always be completely eradicated by the above measures. An alternative, favored by surgeons, but not so many palliative care specialists, is a nasogastric tube aspirated regularly. Some patients may opt for this if offered, others will not.

Emotional Issues

Patients and their families experience a range of emotional problems in coping with this distressing disease. These include anxiety, depression, and anger. Management of these requires a combination of psychological and supportive measures with use of drug treatments as appropriate. Cancer nurse specialists, palliative care nurses, and the patient's primary health care team play key roles in the emotional support of mesothelioma patients and their families, particularly as the condition progresses.

After Death

Where death is thought to have been caused by the patient's occupation, the legal requirements of the particular country must be complied with. In England and Wales, all deaths in which an occupational cause is suspected should be reported to the coroner. Usually a autopsy is performed before an inquest is held, although sometimes the coroner will accept the evidence of a histologically confirmed diagnosis of mesothelioma. Ideally the patient's relatives or carers should have been warned about this in a sensitive manner beforehand. The inquest is usually opened and then adjourned, to allow funeral arrangements. The formal inquest then takes place some months later.

References

1. British Thoracic Society pleural disease guideline 2010. Thorax. 2010;65(Suppl II):4–76.
2. Maskell NA, Butland RJA, on behalf of the British Thoracic Society Pleural Disease Group. BTS guidelines for the investigation of a unilateral pleural effusion in adults. Thorax. 2003;58(Suppl II):ii8–17.
3. Antunes G, Neville E, Duffy J, Ali N, on behalf of the BTS Pleural Disease Group. BTS guidelines for the management of malignant pleural effusions. Thorax. 2003;58(Suppl II):ii29–38.
4. American Thoracic Society. Management of malignant pleural effusions. Am J Respir Crit Care Med. 2000;162:1987–2001.
5. Kolschmann S, Ballin A, Gillissen A. Clinical efficacy and safety of thoracoscopic talc pleurodesis in malignant pleural effusions. Chest. 2005;128:1431–5.
6. Davies HE, Nicholson JE, Rahman NM, Wilkinson EM, Davies RJO, Lee YCG. Outcome of patients with nonspecific pleuritis/fibrosis on thoracoscopic pleural biopsies. Eur J Cardiothorac Surg. 2010;38:472–7.
7. Chapman A, Mulrennan S, Ladd B, Muers MF. Population based epidemiology and prognosis of mesothelioma in Leeds, UK. Thorax. 2008;63:435–9.
8. Musk AW, Olsen N, Alfonso H, et al. Predicting survival in malignant mesothelioma. Eur Respir J. 2011;38:1420–4.
9. Moore S, Darlinson L, Tod AM. Living with mesothelioma. A literature review. Eur J Cancer Care. 2010;19:458–68.
10. British Lung Foundation (BLF) Survey of mesothelioma patients and their carers. London: BLF; 2009.
11. Rakha EA, Patil S, Abdulla K, Abdulkader M, Chaudry Z, Soomro IN. The sensitivity of cytologic evaluation of pleural fluid in the diagnosis of malignant mesothelioma. Diagn Cytopathol. 2010;38:874–9.
12. Edwards JG, Abrams KR, Leverment JN. Prognostic factors for malignant mesothelioma in 142 patients: validation of CALGB and EORTC prognostic scoring systems. Thorax. 2000;55:731–5.
13. Muers MF, Stephens RJ, Fisher P, et al. Active symptom control with or without chemotherapy in the treatment of patients with malignant pleural mesothelioma: results of the Medical Research Council/British Thoracic Society MS01 multi-centre randomised trial (ISRCTN54469112). Lancet. 2008;371:1685–94.
14. Van Meerbeek JP, Gaafar R, Manegold C, et al. A randomised phase III study of cisplatin with or without raltitrexed in patients with malignant pleural mesothelioma: an intergroup study of the European Organisation for Research and Treatment of Cancer Lung Cancer Group and the National Cancer Institute of Canada. J Clin Oncol. 2005;23:6881–9.
15. Vogelzang NJ, Rusthoven JJ, Symanowski J, et al. Phase III study of pemetrexed in combination with cisplatin versus cisplatin alone in patients with malignant pleural mesothelioma. J Clin Oncol. 2003;21:2636–44.
16. O'Brien MER, Watkins Ryan DC. A randomised trial in malignant mesothelioma of early versus delayed chemotherapy in symptomatically stable patients: the MED trial. Ann Oncol. 2006;17:270–5.
17. British Thoracic Society Standards of Care Committee. BTS statement on malignant mesothelioma in the UK. Thorax. 2007;62(Suppl II):1–19.
18. West SD, Foord T, Davies RJO. Needle-track metastases and prophylactic radiotherapy for mesothelioma. Respir Med. 2006;100:1037–40.
19. Chapman E, Garcia Dieguez M. Radiotherapy for malignant pleural mesothelioma (review). The Cochrane Library. 2010:1–12.
20. Hesdorffer ME, Leinwand J, Taub RN. Malignant pleural mesothelioma. J R Coll Physic Edin. 2007;37:232–7.

21. Borasio P, Berruti A, Billé A, et al. Malignant pleural mesothelioma: clinicopathologic and survival characteristics in a consecutive series of 394 patients. Eur J Cardiothorac Surg. 2008;33:307–13.
22. Jackson MB, Pounder D, Price C, Matthews AW, Neville E. Percutaneous cervical cordotomy for the control of pain in patients with pleural mesothelioma. Thorax. 1999;54:238–41.
23. Antrobus JHL, Beaty D. Percutaneous cordotomy. © Mesothelioma UK; 2011.
24. Becker G, Galandi D, Blum HE. Malignant ascites: systemic review and guideline for treatment. Eur J Cancer. 2006;42:589–97.
25. Lee CW, Bociek G, Faught W. A survey of practice in management of malignant ascites. J Pain Symptom Manage. 1998;16:96–101.

Chapter 8
Chronic Obstructive Pulmonary Disease

Graham P. Burns and Rachel Quibell

Abstract Chronic obstructive pulmonary disease (COPD) is one of the commonest causes of death worldwide. It causes substantial disability which progresses over many years. Patients need a high level of treatment and supportive care throughout the course of the disease. A key goal of treatment is to improve patient-centered outcomes such as quality of life, symptom burden, and the impact of symptoms on the patient's overall functioning. Palliative care of COPD is particularly complex because of the clinical course of the disease over many years, the unpredictable trajectory of the disease and the fact that patients often die from other causes. End of life issues and anticipatory care planning should be discussed in patients with advanced COPD but disease-specific therapies, emergency management of exacerbations, and palliative supportive care must run in parallel in an integrated manner. The dying phase is often short, over a few days, when the patient fails to recover from the final exacerbation.

Keywords Chronic obstructive pulmonary disease • Non-invasive ventilation Mechanical ventilation • Pulmonary rehabilitation • Oxygen • Breathlessness

Chronic obstructive pulmonary disease (COPD) is the preferred term for the constellation of respiratory conditions associated with cigarette smoking, principally chronic bronchitis and emphysema. It represents an enormous burden of disease on a global scale. In the UK, an estimated three million people have the disease (though only about 900,000 are diagnosed) [1]. By 2020 the World Health Organization

G.P. Burns, B.Sc., M.B.B.S., FRCP, DipMedSci., Ph.D. (✉)
Department of Respiratory Medicine, Royal Victoria Infirmary,
Queen Victoria Road, Newcastle upon Tyne NE1 4LP, UK
e-mail: graham.burns@nuth.nhs.uk

R. Quibell, M.B.B.S., FRCP
Department of Palliative Medicine, Royal Victoria Infirmary,
Newcastle upon Tyne, UK

S.J. Bourke, E.T. Peel (eds.), *Integrated Palliative Care of Respiratory Disease*,
DOI 10.1007/978-1-4471-2230-2_8, © Springer-Verlag London 2013

expects it to be the third biggest cause of death worldwide. In the UK, there are about 110,000 admissions to hospital and 30,000 deaths each year from COPD. At an individual level, there is a wide spectrum of severity, although it often causes substantial, progressive disability and significant impairment of quality of life.

Chronic bronchitis is caused by mucus hypersecretion and is manifest as chronic cough and sputum production. Emphysema and the associated airway obstruction lead to gradually progressive breathlessness. Because of large respiratory reserve, patients with a sedentary lifestyle often do not notice breathlessness until a great deal of lung function has been permanently lost. Most patients are not diagnosed until they are in their 50s when the disease can be at an advanced stage. The disease course of gradual progressive breathlessness and disability is punctuated by episodes of an acute worsening of symptoms, usually associated with infection. These exacerbations tend to occur with increasing frequency and severity as the disease progresses. In advanced disease, they are accompanied by breathlessness at rest, often necessitate hospital admission, and can be life threatening.

There is now increasing recognition of the importance of the non-respiratory manifestations of COPD. These result, in part, from the deconditioning associated with disability though also, to some extent, from the systemic "overspill" of the inflammatory mediators. They include fatigue, malaise, muscle wasting, reduced appetite, weight loss, osteoporosis, anxiety and depression. Good quality, holistic care of COPD should address all aspects of the condition and not merely focus on treatments aimed at improving airway obstruction.

Palliative Care in COPD

Providing palliative care to patients with COPD is complex, and sometimes contentious, because of the clinical course of the disease over many years, the unpredictable trajectory of dying, and the fact that patients often die from other causes, rather than from their COPD. The disease is typically characterized by a very long phase of disability during which patients and their families need a high level of treatment and supportive care. During this phase, patients have substantial symptoms which need to be addressed with a holistic comprehensive approach. As the disease progresses, patients often need frequent admissions to hospital for exacerbations which result in severe acute symptoms and distress and which significantly impair their quality of life. End of life issues and anticipatory care planning may be discussed over a period of time during the advanced stage of the disease, but the dying phase is often quite short, over a few days, when patients fail to recover from their final exacerbation. Clinicians are often surprised at how long a patient may live despite having very advanced disease, and paradoxically the patient, family, and clinical team can also be taken by surprise when the patient eventually dies since recovery has been the outcome of many previous crises. It is clear that some traditional models of provision of palliative care, often based on the cancer trajectory, do not suit patients with chronic lung diseases such COPD. In this setting, much of the ongoing palliative and supportive care is delivered by a multidisciplinary respiratory team. There is a crucial role for palliative care specialists in the education of respiratory teams in the skills and ethos of palliation. A key goal of treatment is to improve patient-centered outcomes, such as quality of life, symptom burden, and the impact of symptoms on the patient's overall functioning, with less reliance on the more traditional outcome measures such as change in lung function tests. Considerable progress has been made in achieving holistic patient-centered care for these patients, with more provision of care at home, and better coordination of services across the primary and secondary care sectors in hospital and in the community. For these patients it is clear that palliative care, disease-specific treatments, symptom-control measures, supportive care, emergency care, palliative care, and end of life care must run in parallel throughout the course of the disease. Specialist palliative care teams play a particular role at certain stages of the disease. They can support the respiratory team in dealing with distressing and disabling symptoms at any stage of the disease. As the disease progresses they can facilitate discussions about the patient's wishes, hopes, and expectations about future care. This is discussed further in Chap. 13, using COPD as an example of anticipatory and advanced care planning. End of life care for patients dying from COPD often occurs in the context of an acute exacerbation which has failed to respond to treatment. It is important that intensive treatment of the exacerbation should also focus on management of the patient's symptoms and on relief of distress. When it is clear that the patient has failed to respond to treatment of the exacerbation and is now dying, the focus of care transitions to managing the dying phase using an integrated care pathway such as the Liverpool care pathway for the dying patient. Specialist palliative care services may be able to facilitate a patient's wish to be at home when dying, and to help the family cope with the final illness and bereavement phase.

COPD produces a symptom burden which is often greater than that experienced by many cancer patients, yet historically COPD patients have not benefited from specialist palliative care services to the same extent as cancer patients [2]. The argument that they should has been made with some conviction in recent years. However, the needs of patients with COPD differ significantly from those with cancer and the best way of providing on-going palliative and supportive care throughout the long course of the disease has not yet been fully established [3]. Unlike cancer, there is no clear distinction between the disease-specific and palliative phases of treatment. In COPD life expectancy is usually many years; treatment is therefore very much about enhancing quality of life, rather than managing an inevitable decline to death. Care should be based on need and symptoms rather than prognosis. Most care is provided by the multidisciplinary respiratory team using the principles of general palliative care, supported by specialist palliative care teams in an integrated fashion, working alongside the respiratory team in order to identify patients with needs for specialist input in symptom-management or in addressing end of life issues as the disease progresses. Many respiratory units already deliver a holistic approach with a team of healthcare specialists offering a broad range of effective interventions, including smoking cessation support, pharmacological management of breathlessness, cough and exacerbations, physiotherapy for airway clearance, patient education, pulmonary rehabilitation for cardiovascular de-conditioning, and cognitive behavioral therapy for anxiety and depression. The expertise of the palliative care specialist should be integral to that holistic approach and is invaluable in complex patients, irrespective of the stage of their disease.

In the dying phase when the downward trajectory to death becomes inevitable and relatively predictable, the aims and focus of treatment clearly change. In this context, the specialist skills of the palliative care specialist may come to the fore. Because of the nature of the condition, however, in most cases death only becomes firmly predictable in the last few hours of life. Typically a formal decision to focus on providing comfort care in the dying phase is made when attempts at prolonging life have clearly failed. This is often in hospital after an intense period of active treatment perhaps including non-invasive ventilation. In such circumstances, when death finally intervenes, one is apt to reflect and, with genuine compassion, question whether the outcome should have been foreseen and a less aggressive, more symptom-focused approach adopted sooner. The question is eminently reasonable, the answer not always straightforward.

Can We Predict Survival in the Stable Phase of the Disease?

COPD is generally regarded as being associated with a poor prognosis. Many health care professionals managing patients with COPD however might be surprised to know that most people with COPD do not actually die from COPD. In the TORCH study, around 6,000 patients with a forced expiratory volume in one second (FEV1)<60 % predicted were followed up for a 3 year period to observe the effect of various inhaler treatments on all-cause mortality [4]. Overall the probability of death from any cause at 3 years was only around 14 %. Of the deaths that occurred a minority, only 30 %, were COPD-related. Other common causes of death included cardiovascular disease and cancer. In fact in the maximally treated group (on salmeterol and fluticasone propionate combination inhaler), the probability of death from any cause at 3 years was reduced to 12.6 % and the probability of COPD-related death was only 4.7 %.

It may seem reasonable to assume that in more advanced disease (lower FEV1) survival will be worse. In a study by Celli et al. however, FEV1 was not a strong predictor of mortality [5]. Celli identified four variables: body-mass index (B), degree of airflow obstruction (O), dyspnea (D), and exercise capacity (E), which when combined in a multidimensional 10-point scale (the BODE index) proved to be much better at predicting mortality over the 52 month follow up. When the BODE score was divided in quartiles, the highest quartile (BODE 7–10) had a survival of around 20 % after 52 months of follow-up compared with a survival of around 80 % in the lowest quartile (BODE 0–2). Nevertheless, it should be noted that even the patients in the worst quartile were more likely to be alive after 3 years than not. Prognosis is difficult to predict accurately in individual patients and most patients will die of something other than COPD. Patients, their families, and their clinical teams often have to live with the uncertainty of the prognosis.

Can We Predict Survival in the Acute Phase of the Disease?

The disease course in COPD is characterized by a relatively constant level of disability interspersed by less predictable exacerbations. Some exacerbations are severe enough to warrant admission to hospital and are, in a very real sense, life threatening. Can we be more confident about predicting survival in this acute context? In patients admitted to hospital with exacerbations of COPD, the group who develop acute acidotic respiratory failure (pH < 7.35) have, by far, the greatest risk of death. In this context, non-invasive ventilation (NIV) is known to be an effective therapy. In the seminal work on the use of NIV in a real world setting, Plant et al. found the introduction of NIV, early after the admission on a general respiratory ward, was effective at reducing the risk of death and the need for endotracheal intubation and mechanical ventilation in an intensive care unit (ICU) [6]. In patients admitted with a pH in the range 7.25–7.35, in-patient mortality in those receiving "standard therapy" was 20 %; this was reduced to 10 % in those given NIV. Clearly when treatment with NIV offers a 50 % reduction in the risk of death and with a probability of survival of 90 %, most patients would opt to have this treatment, and emergency admission to hospital would be appropriate. In the ISIS2 study, the first trial that identified survival advantage of thrombolysis in the context of acute myocardial infarction, the improvement in mortality was only 40 %. Yet it in this context, this was quickly established as standard treatment [7].

In a national UK audit of clinical care of 9,716 patients admitted with COPD, management tended to be far more conservative than the evidence would suggest it should be: 30 % of those with persisting acidosis did not receive NIV [8]. Of those who did receive NIV, 55 % had a pH < 7.25 in which context endotracheal intubation and ventilation in an ICU is likely to have offered a greater chance of survival. In a real-life retrospective analysis of survival in patients receiving NIV, similar deficiencies in management were identified [9]. However in follow up after discharge, 70 % of patients were still alive 1 year later. Therefore, it would seem that if the optimal care identified in studies could be offered to those patients presenting in acute respiratory failure then the vast majority would not only survive to discharge but still be alive 1 year later.

A particularly difficult issue in the management of advanced COPD is whether endotracheal intubation and mechanical ventilation in an ICU is an appropriate treatment option for some patients [10]. This is discussed further in Chap. 12. Appropriately selected patients certainly benefit from admission to ICU with endotracheal intubation and mechanical ventilation. A long-term retrospective analysis of COPD patients (mean FEV1 0.74L) in acute respiratory failure managed with mechanical ventilation showed that 79.7 % were successfully weaned and survived to discharge from hospital [11]. The median duration of ventilation was 2 days and only 13 % received ventilatory support for more than 1 week. Parameters such as FEV1, functional performance scores, or the use of long-term oxygen therapy prior to admission were not significant determinants of long-term survival. The presence of comorbidities, however, significantly affected survival. In another large retrospective series, 72 % of those ventilated survived weaning to discharge, in patients without comorbidities that figure rose to 88 % [12]. It has also been shown in a prospective study that the presence of non-respiratory organ failure was the most significant predictor of both in-hospital and 6-month survival [13].

It would seem that survival, even in the context of a severe exacerbation with respiratory failure, is probably better than many clinicians would estimate. It would also appear to be very difficult to predict in an individual patient. This lack of certainty, of course, should not preclude an integrated approach to care, with specialist palliative input based on need rather than assumed prognosis. A holistic assessment of spiritual, emotional, and physical needs and the balancing of benefit and burden can take place in the context of uncertainty and ongoing active management. Prognostic uncertainty should never be an excuse for denying good supportive and specialist palliative care if needed. Both active and palliative care can work in parallel to the benefit of patients.

Advance Care Planning and End of Life Discussions

In 2009, a qualitative study of health care professionals looking at barriers to advance care planning (ACP) in COPD revealed "inadequate information provision about the likely course of COPD at diagnosis" and a "lack of consensus in relation to initiating ACP" [14]. Recent initiatives emphasize the benefits of anticipatory and advance care planning, and discussions about end of life issues, in patients with advanced stage disease [15]. However, considerable difficulties are encountered when this approach is applied in practice and it is clear that there are some limitations to advanced care planning when an uncertain disease trajectory is inherent to the disease, when the patient may live many years with significant disability, and ultimately die from another cause [16]. Clinicians and services must adapt to this uncertainty. It can be unhelpful and often inappropriate to try to predict prognosis accurately; rather it is necessary to plan for what the patient may wish to happen under certain circumstances which may arise.

The distressing symptoms and physical limitations that come with COPD have, in themselves, a major negative psychological impact. Depression is common. Patients "give up" and avoid a number of activities that their physical condition would not absolutely preclude. One of the aims of good COPD care is to empower and enable patients; to change the mindset from one of "life is over" to a more positive outlook where activity, function, and quality of life are maximized. Undue focus on "inevitable mortality" can be distressing and often inappropriate for many of these patients. In a study which set out to examine the barriers to end of life care communication for patients with oxygen dependant COPD, 115 patients were interviewed by trained research interviewers [17]. Rather than a lack of opportunity or apparent unwillingness on the part of their physician, the barrier to such discussions most commonly cited by the patients was: "I'd rather concentrate on staying alive."

Anticipatory management plans formulated by clinical teams and advanced care plans devised by patients need to be adapted over the course of time. When an acute crisis develops, what had seemed reasonable in discussion a year earlier is often at odds with the immediate choices a patient might now make? In general, surveys most people say that they would (some day) like to die at home, surrounded by their family, not in pain. In a crisis, even in the context of a known terminal illness, those same individuals often chose the comfort and security of hospital. This should not necessarily be seen as a deficiency in medical services to deliver what patients really want but a reflection of the distinction between an abstract wish about the future and a choice made in the face of an acute exacerbation provoking a high level of symptoms and distress. In the context of an exacerbation of COPD, there is the additional expectation of treatment that will make them well again. Urgent assessment and intervention can bring symptom relief and control of a distressing crisis, and can allow a decision to be made with the patient and family on the best course of action at that time.

Perhaps the most appropriate and indeed productive time to initiate a discussion about end of life issues is an outpatient visit following an admission with life-threatening respiratory failure in which NIV was used. In this context, about 30 % of patients would be expected to die over the coming year. A discussion about preferences for treatment in the event of a similar episode in future, at the very least, has clear meaning to the patient. The conversation could then focus, for example, on whether, given similar circumstances, they would wish to have NIV treatment again, balancing the benefit and burden of treatment. Following such an unhurried, fully informed discussion, away from the fog of the acute crisis the decision reached by the patient would seem to be the best possible representation of their true wishes.

If, some 6 months later, the patient were re-admitted in need of NIV, of course the decision would be reviewed. The patient should not feel bound by any earlier "decision." The problem with discussions away from the acute situation is that in the next acute crisis the patient may have changed their mind. This is an inherent challenge in advance care planning and advanced decisions to refuse treatment, and is discussed in greater detail in Chap. 13.

When doctors make decisions on the appropriateness of withholding treatment, they are influenced by what they believe to be fairly objective assessments of the patient's global quality of life, physical comfort, mobility, and depression [18]. Critically however, the doctor's estimate tends to be worse than the patients' own estimate of their quality of life. Perhaps doctors are influenced by how they imagine they would view things if suddenly confronted by the predicament the patient finds himself in. Trying to second guess a patient's wishes makes little sense. It is no substitute for open communication. We also need to remain acutely aware of how much we influence the decisions of our patients and we must strive to be as balanced as possible in such discussions. When doctors and patient open up the communication channels, it is often the doctor who learns more. "Natural assumptions" about what the patient may think or be concerned about are often wrong. It may well be that mortality per se is not the issue. A common overriding fear is of dying of breathlessness or "suffocation." Once the concern is understood, some re-assurance can often be offered. Perhaps the best way forward is to establish a rapport between physician and patient that allows regular open discussion of the individual patient's hopes and expectations as well as fears in relation to symptom control and evolving end of life care.

This would form the basis of an effective integrated palliative care approach focusing on quality of life at all stages. For many this broader approach may be more appropriate and more productive than focusing primarily on death [19]. There are some patients however who want to have conversations around specific end of life issues and wish to make advanced directives. We need to be receptive and be led by our patients' wishes.

Symptomatic Control

Dyspnea

Much of the management of COPD, from the time of diagnosis until death, is about the palliation of dyspnea. Dyspnea in COPD is driven largely by the mechanisms that relate to airway obstruction and the resulting hyperinflation. These are discussed in detail in Chap. 2. Anxiety is a very common accompaniment; triggered by breathlessness but also providing a positive feedback loop augmenting both the sensation and its unpleasantness.

Pharmacological Management

Bronchodilatation

As airflow obstruction is the cardinal feature of COPD, bronchodilatation is the first-pharmacological intervention to alleviate breathlessness. Bronchodilators fall into two categories; those that stimulate the sympathetic pathways, beta-2 agonists, and those that block the parasympathetic pathways, the anticholinergics. In each of these groups, there are short-acting and long-acting drugs.

Salbutamol is the most commonly used bronchodilator; it is a short-acting beta-2 agonist. It can be delivered via an inhaler which is convenient for portable everyday use. Its quick onset of action, though short duration of effect makes it ideal as an "as required reliever." Some degree of maintenance bronchodilatation can be achieved by long-acting beta agonists such as formoterol or salmeterol whose duration of action is around 12 h. More recently, a longer acting (24 h) beta agonist, indacaterol, has become available [20]. Any one of these long-acting agents can be used in conjunction with salbutamol to achieve and maintain maximum beta agonist stimulation. When patients are severely unwell and hospital admission is required, they may need higher doses than can be easily delivered by an inhaler. Under these circumstances, it is reasonable to use the drug via nebulization. For longer term (chronic) management however, maximum bronchodilatation can be achieved by correct use of an inhaler and there is generally no place for home nebulizer use in long-term management. Ipratropium bromide is a short-acting anticholinergic bronchodilator. As it acts via a different mechanism to salbutamol, the two drugs can be used together with an effect above and beyond what either agent would deliver alone. Nebulized ipratropium is still commonly used in situations when nebulizer therapy is necessary. In its inhaler form ipratropium has been superseded by tiotropium, a long-acting anticholinergic bronchodilator. This is not only more convenient (in its once daily dose regimen) but also, even when compared with four times per day ipratropium, it is a better bronchodilator, it is better at improving both dyspnea and quality of life scores. Unfortunately, unlike the beta agonists, the long- and short-acting anticholinergics cannot be used in conjunction with each other; they tend to lead to unwanted anticholinergic side effects such as dry mouth and blurred vision.

Oxygen

Understandably many patients (and their families) believe that the best treatment for breathlessness is oxygen. However, it is crucial for healthcare professionals to understand that a patient "short of breath" is not necessarily "short of oxygen," and that oxygen therapy is not indicated unless the patient is hypoxemic [21]. In prospective double-blind, randomized controlled trials of breathlessness, oxygen showed no benefit in alleviating dyspnea in patients without hypoxemia [22]. Only hypoxic patients may derive benefit. In considering the appropriateness of oxygen prescription, it is also important to remain mindful of its significant drawbacks: restriction of activities, possible impairment of quality of life, and psychological dependence.

In the UK, there are three modalities of home oxygen delivery [21]: (1) Long-term oxygen therapy, which is proven to reduce mortality in carefully selected patients. (2) Ambulatory oxygen, which can improve exercise tolerance and quality of life in carefully selected patients. (3) Short burst oxygen therapy, which is the only modality in which the indication is ill-defined and which has no formal assessment criteria.

Opioids

Used systemically in the acute setting opioids have an important role in relieving breathlessness [23]. Their use is discussed in more detail in Chap. 2. Studies that have examined the effect of nebulized opioids on breathlessness in respiratory disease have consistently demonstrated that they are no more effective than nebulized saline [23]. This is probably because the afferent signals which inform the sensation of breathlessness in the advanced stages of COPD do not originate within the airways.

Non-pharmacological Management

Anxiety Management

Anxiety as an issue in its own right is discussed below. Its link with breathlessness however is an intimate one with a two-way causal relationship. When dealing with breathlessness at any stage of COPD, including very advanced disease, "think anxiety." It can, otherwise, easily be overlooked.

Pulmonary Rehabilitation

Pulmonary rehabilitation is a multidisciplinary programme of care for patients with chronic respiratory impairment. It comprises individualized exercise programmes and educational talks which aim to prevent de-conditioning and allow the patient to cope with their disease. It is an effective treatment for patients from moderate to severe COPD and is proven to lead to statistically significant and clinically mean-ingful improvements in dyspnea, exercise capacity, and health-related quality of life. Though clearly not appropriate for true end of life care, it should not be overlooked as an effective addition to management even in advanced disease.

Other Non-pharmacological Management

A Cochrane review examined a number of other non-pharmacological strategies and techniques tried for the alleviation of breathlessness [24]. These are discussed in detail in Chap. 2.

Symptoms Other Than Breathlessness

Anxiety and Depression

There is little in the realm of human experience more frightening than not being able to breathe. In severe attacks of breathlessness, patients often report that they feel as if they are going to die. Clearly when such attacks become a frequent, though unpredictable, part of life, they are apt to render even the most psychologically robust individual rather anxious. COPD is characterized by episodes of severe breathlessness. Though anxiety may be a normal human response to such attacks, it is not a helpful one. Breathlessness leads to anxiety, which leads to an increased respiratory rate and heightens the sense of breathlessness, thereby fueling anxiety in a vicious cycle. On occasions this spirals out of control into a full blown "panic attack." Panic disorder is up to ten times more prevalent in patients with COPD than in the general population [25].

COPD brings physical limitation to life's activities. Patients note a gradual contrac-tion of their world. At some point their ability to walk around town is lost, not long after that they find they are unable to get to the corner shop, soon the garden gate is the limit of their world and finally they are unable to get beyond their own front door. They become isolated. They cease to take part in life. "Life" is then what other people walking past the window do. Depression is common in COPD. Perhaps the only surprising feature is that it seems to be just as common in mild as in severe disease.

In our unit we recently investigated a stable outpatient COPD population. One-hundred and ninety-six patients were screened using the Hospital Anxiety and Depression (HAD) questionnaire over a 6-month period. We found 78 % of patients had anxiety and 55 % of patients had depression (respective scores ≥8). There were no significant associations with COPD NICE severity stage or gender.

Anxiety and depression are critically important issues in their own right and worthy targets of treatment in COPD. But their impact on the individual extends beyond the purely psychological. Whilst breathlessness itself leads to avoidance of physical activity, which in turn leads to de-conditioning and increased breathlessness, the fear and frustration so common in COPD leads to other inappropriate avoidance (such as a reluctance to participate in pulmonary rehabilitation) and safety-seeking behaviour such as inappropriate presentation to emergency services. Anxiety is a significant predictor of the frequency of hospital admissions and re-admissions for acute exacerbations of COPD [25]. In COPD, depression has an effect on smoking status, symptom burden and physical functioning and even rates of admission to hospital [26].

Identifying anxiety and depression is a necessary step in providing support for patients. As many of the symptoms of anxiety (such as breathlessness) and depression (such as fatigue) overlap with the symptoms of COPD, recognition of the problem can be difficult. Formal screening using tools such as the Hospital Anxiety and Depression questionnaire should be a routine part of practice. Once identified, anxiety and depression should be addressed just as conscientiously as airway obstruction. This rarely occurs [2]. The reasons for this are complex. It is often thought that patients might misunderstand the focus on anxiety and panic as a suggestion that their symptoms are not "real" or that they may be resistant to acknowledging the problem because of the stigma associated with mental illness [27]. Experience suggests this is rarely the case. Once given the opportunity to discuss anxiety, panic, and depression, patients often feel a great sense of release and are not only keen to open up and discuss these issues but are very amenable to accepting treatment. It remains true however that many health professionals feel ill-equipped to deal with psychological issues and the dominant medical model culture results in very little attention being paid to the patient's psychological well-being.

In the management of anxiety and depression patients should have access to psychological treatments, pharmacological treatments, or both in combination [1]. Cognitive behavioral therapy (CBT) is a psychological "talking" treatment which explores the links between situations thoughts, feelings, physical symptoms, and behavior. Unhelpful thoughts and behavior can be challenged and changed. In coming to understand these links, patients develop new skills and can, in the longer term, effectively act as their own therapists. Patients are empowered. Learning to address psychological problems can be empowering for the healthcare professional also. Access to trained therapists remains a stumbling block. However, healthcare professionals, such as respiratory nurse specialists, can be trained in CBT skills and can apply these usefully in their day to day practice.

Fatigue

Fatigue is a complex issue and a common symptom in many advanced diseases. In the context of advanced COPD, the factors contributing to the sensation are most likely to be breathlessness, depression, and de-conditioning; each of which may be identifiable and amenable to treatment as discussed above. There is also increasing evidence that COPD is a systemic condition [28]. "Spill-over" of inflammatory mediators into the circulation can result in systemic manifestations of the disease, such as muscle wasting and cachexia which can also contribute to the sense of "fatigue." Research to better understand this systemic component of COPD, and hopefully manage it, is ongoing. Until specific remedies are developed, it is at least useful to recognize its existence. Nutritional supplements may offer some support.

Xerostomia

Xerostomia (dryness of the mouth) is commonly reported in the advanced stages of COPD. Potential factors contributing to the condition include side effect of treatment (e.g., anticholinergic and opioids), mouth breathing, non-humidified oxygen, dehydration, candidiasis, anxiety, and depression. Any one or any combination of these factors may be present in advanced COPD. Identification of the contributory factors should assist with management as most can be modulated. Other general measures include frequent sips of (ice cold) water, and stimulation of the production of saliva using, for example, chewing gum, acid drops, lemon drinks, and sucking ice cubes.

Cough

Cough is a very common symptom in COPD in general. Chronic bronchitis (persistent productive cough) is the facet of COPD that can improve or even resolve on smoking cessation. Resolution however tends to take a month or two as the awakened airway cilia set about clearing the accumulated excess airway mucus. After smoking cessation, unless the patient has co-existing bronchiectasis, productive cough more commonly tends to be restricted to periods of "exacerbation" (which are usually, though not always, associated with infection). These usually respond to courses of antibiotics and steroids. When exacerbations are frequent, regular inhaled tiotropium and combination inhalers, such as fluticasone and salmeterol or budesonide and formoterol, twice a day can significantly reduce the exacerbation rate. Although, as yet less well established, thrice weekly azithromycin 250 mg also seems to be effective when exacerbations are very frequent [29]. In the context of severe disease (FEV1 <50 % predicted), chronic productive cough can be improved by roflumilast, through in the UK the National Institute for Clinical Excellence (NICE) did not find this to be a cost-effective treatment for general use [30].

Organization of Integrated Palliative Care in COPD

Palliative care of COPD is complex and the best way of planning care for these patients has not yet been fully established. It is unlikely that one model of palliative care will suit all patients and considerable flexibility is needed in order to meet the complex needs of these patients [3]. Because of the trajectory of the disease over many years, it is apparent that disease-specific care, supportive care, emergency care, palliative care, and end of life care must run in parallel, and that a division between active and palliative care is artificial and not usually appropriate for these patients. The emphasis on different aspects of care will change as the disease progresses. Most care will be general palliative and supportive care delivered by the holistic respiratory multidisciplinary team using general palliative principles but there is an important and increasing role for input and support from specialist palliative medicine teams. This includes a role in the education and support of the respiratory team in the knowledge, skills, and ethos of palliative care. Specialist palliative care clinicians, working as part of the wider multidisciplinary respiratory team, can identify patients with particular needs requiring specialist palliative care input, assist with anticipatory care planning, enable patients to be at home when dying if that is their wish, and support families during the dying phase and during bereavement.

References

1. National Institute for Health and Clinical Excellence (NICE). Management of chronic obstructive pulmonary disease in adults in primary and secondary care (partial update). Clinical guidelines CG101 Issued. 2010. http://guidance.nice.org.uk/CG101. Accessed Apr 2012.
2. Gore JM, Brophy CJ, Greenstone MA. How well do we care for patients with end stage chronic obstructive pulmonary disease (COPD)? A comparison of palliative care and quality of life in COPD and lung cancer. Thorax. 2000;55:1000–6.
3. Lanken PN, Terry PB, DeLisser HM, et al. An official American Thoracic Society clinical policy statement: palliative care for patients with respiratory diseases and critical illnesses. Am J Respir Crit Care Med. 2008;177:912–27.
4. Calverley PMA, Anderson JA, Celli B et al. for the TORCH investigators. Salmeterol and fluticasone propionate and survival in chronic obstructive pulmonary disease. N Engl J Med. 2007;356:775–89.
5. Celli BR, Cote CG, Marin JM, et al. The body-mass index, airflow obstruction, dyspnea, and exercise capacity index in chronic obstructive pulmonary disease. N Engl J Med. 2004;350:1005–12.
6. Plant PK, Owen JL, Elliott MW. Early use of non-invasive ventilation for acute exacerbations of chronic obstructive pulmonary disease on general respiratory wards: a multicentre randomised controlled trial. Lancet. 2000;355:1931–5.
7. Randomised trial of intravenous streptokinase, oral aspirin, both, or neither among 17,187 cases of suspected acute myocardial infarction: ISIS-2. ISIS-2 (Second International Study of Infarct Survival) Collaborative Group. Lancet. 1988;2:349–60.
8. Roberts CM, Stone RA, Buckingham RJ, Pursey NA, Lowe D. Acidosis, non-invasive ventilation and mortality in hospitalised COPD exacerbations. Thorax. 2011;66:43–8.
9. Murray I, Paterson E, Thain G, Currie GP. Outcomes following non-invasive ventilation for hypercapnic exacerbations of chronic obstructive pulmonary disease. Thorax. 2011;66:825–6.

10. Simmonds AK. Ethics and decision making in end stage lung disease. Thorax. 2003;58:272–7.
11. Breen D, Churches T, Hawker F, Torzillo PJ. Acute respiratory failure secondary to chronic obstructive pulmonary disease treated in the intensive care unit: a long term follow up study. Thorax. 2002;57:29–33.
12. Nevins ML, Epstein SK. Predictors of outcome for patients with COPD requiring invasive mechanical ventilation. Chest. 2001;119:1840–9.
13. Seneff MG, Wagner DP, Wagner RP, Zimmerman JE, Knaus WA. Hospital and 1-year survival of patients admitted to intensive care units with acute exacerbation of chronic obstructive pulmonary disease. JAMA. 1995;274:1852–7.
14. Gott M, Gardiner C, Small N, et al. Barriers to advance care planning in chronic obstructive pulmonary disease. Palliat Med. 2009;23:642–8.
15. Richards M. End of life care strategy. London: Department of Health; 2008. www.dh.gov.uk/en/Healthcare/IntegratedCare/Endoflifecare/index.htm. Accessed Apr 2012.
16. Reinke LF, Slatore CG, Uman J, et al. Patient-clinician communication about end of life care topics: is anyone talking to patients with chronic obstructive pulmonary disease? J Palliat Med. 2011;14:923–8.
17. Knauft E, Nielsen EL, Engelberg RA, Patrick DL, Curtis JR. Barriers and facilitators to end of life care communication for patients with COPD. Chest. 2005;127:2188–96.
18. Golin CE, Wenger NS, Liu H, et al. A prospective study of patient-physician communication about resuscitation. J Am Geriatr Soc. 2000;48(Suppl):S52–60.
19. Hill AT, Hopkinson RB, Stableforth DE. Ventilation in a Birmingham intensive care unit 1993–1995: outcome for patients with chronic obstructive pulmonary disease. Respir Med. 1999;92:156–61.
20. Mahler DA, D'Urzo A, Bateman ED, et al. Concurrent use of indacaterol plus tiotropium in patients with COPD provides superior bronchodilation compared with tiotropium alone: a randomised, double-blind comparison. Thorax. 2012. doi:10.1136/thoraxjnl-2011-201140.
21. Gibson GJ. Oxygen treatment at home. BMJ. 2006;332:191.
22. Abernethy AP, McDonald CF, Frith PA, et al. Effect of palliative oxygen versus room air in relief of breathlessness in patients with refractory dyspnoea: a double-blind, randomised controlled trial. Lancet. 2010;376:784–93.
23. Ben-Aharon I, Gafter-Gvili A, Paul M, Leibovici L, Stemmer SM. Interventions for alleviating cancer-related dyspnoea: a systematic review. J Clin Oncol. 2008;26:2396–404.
24. Bauswein C, Booth S, Gysels M, Higginson I. Non-pharmacological interventions for breathlessness in advanced stages of malignant and non-malignant diseases. Cochrane Database Syst Rev. 2008;(2):CD005623.
25. Yohannes AM, Baldwin RC, Connolly MJ. Depression and anxiety in elderly outpatients with chronic obstructive pulmonary disease: prevalence, and validation of the BASDEC screening questionnaire. Int J Geriatr Psychiatry. 2000;15:1090–6.
26. Ng TP, Niti M, Tan WC, Cao Z, Ong KC, Eng P. Depressive symptoms and chronic obstructive pulmonary disease: effect on mortality, hospital readmission, symptom burden, functional status, and quality of life. Arch Intern Med. 2007;167:60–7.
27. Yellowlees PM, Haynes S, Potts N, Ruffin RE. Psychiatric morbidity in patients with life-threatening asthma: initial report of a controlled study. Med J Aust. 1988;149:246–9.
28. Nussbaumer-Ochsner Y, Rabe KF. Systemic manifestations of COPD. Chest. 2011;139:165–73.
29. Albert RK, Connett J, Bailey WC, et al. Azithromycin for prevention of exacerbations of COPD. N Engl J Med. 2011;365:689–98.
30. National Institute for Health and Clinical Excellence. Roflumilast for the management of severe chronic obstructive pulmonary disease. NICE technology appraisal guidance 244. 2012. www.nice.org.uk/ta244. Accessed Apr 2012.

Chapter 9
Interstitial Lung Disease

Ian A. Forrest and E. Timothy Peel

Abstract The term interstitial lung disease covers a number of conditions affecting the interstitium of the lung. The commonest of these is idiopathic pulmonary fibrosis (IPF). IPF usually presents with breathlessness and/or cough. The three pillars of care management strategy includes (1) disease-centered management, (2) symptom-centered management, and (3) education and self-management. Sadly there is no strong evidence of any beneficial drug treatment on the natural history of IPF, although oxygen and lung transplant may both have a role. The symptomatic management of breathlessness and cough, as well as the other symptoms of more advanced disease, is considered in other chapters. The chapter concludes with a ten-point approach to the palliative management of IPF patients.

Keywords Idiopathic pulmonary fibrosis • Disease management • Symptom management • Self management • Breathlessness • Cough

I.A. Forrest, B.Sc., M.B., ChB., Ph.D., FRCP
Department of Respiratory Medicine, Royal Victoria Infirmary, Newcastle upon Tyne, UK

E.T. Peel, M.B.B.S., B.Sc., FRCP(✉)
Department of Palliative Medicine, North Tyneside General Hospital,
Rake Lane, North Shields, Tyne and Wear NE29 8NH, UK

Marie Curie Hospice,
Newcastle upon Tyne, UK
e-mail: tim.peel@northumbria-healthcare.nhs.uk

S.J. Bourke, E.T. Peel (eds.), *Integrated Palliative Care of Respiratory Disease*, 143
DOI 10.1007/978-1-4471-2230-2_9, © Springer-Verlag London 2013

Background

Interstitial lung disease (ILD), sometimes also described as diffuse parenchymal lung disease, refers to a diverse range of over 200 different disease entities that affect the alveoli, distal airways, and interstitium of the lung. The pathology of ILD is characterized by inflammation and fibrosis, often co-existing and commonly resulting in chronic progressive lung disease with substantial morbidity and significant mortality. The classification of ILD is complex and confusing, partly because of variable terminology, historical descriptors, and international differences in nomenclature [1]. The diagnosis of ILD relies on careful integration of clinical features, radiology, and, in a subgroup of patients, histopathological findings in a multidisciplinary approach to these challenging diseases [2]. International guidelines have attempted to classify the ILDs and a useful working classification, which helps inform prognosis and treatment decisions, is outlined in Fig. 9.1 [3].

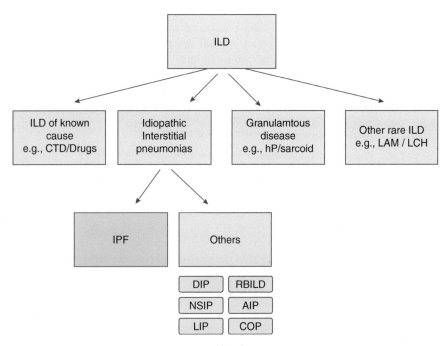

Fig. 9.1 Classification of interstitial lung disease (*ILD*). Idiopathic pulmonary fibrosis (*IPF*) is the most common idiopathic interstitial pneumonia (*IIP*) and is the archetypal fibrotic lung disease. All ILDs however can result in progressive fibrotic lung disease, worsening symptoms, impaired gas exchange, and ultimately death (The figure describes a classification of ILD adapted from the 2002 international consensus [3]). *CTD* connective tissue disease, *HP* hypersensitivity pneumonitis, *LAM* lymphangioleiomyomatosis, *LCH* Langerhans cell histiocytosis, *DIP* desquamative interstitial pneumonia, *NSIP* non specific interstitial pneumonia, *LIP* lymphoid interstitial pneumonia, *RBILD* respiratory bronchiolitis ILD, *AIP* acute interstitial pneumonia, *COP* cryptogenic organizing pneumonia

Many forms of ILD are idiopathic, where no etiological factors can be identified, whereas others are clearly linked to connective tissue diseases, prescribed drugs, cigarette smoking, and environmental exposures to antigens or dusts. The most common ILDs are idiopathic pulmonary fibrosis (IPF) and other idiopathic interstitial pneumonias (IIPs), sarcoidosis, connective tissue disease-associated ILD, and hypersensitivity pneumonitis (also known as extrinsic allergic alveolitis).

Interstitial lung diseases commonly present with dry cough and breathlessness. Examination findings may confirm finger clubbing and crackles on auscultation whilst chest radiography may show diffuse abnormalities including infiltrates, fibrosis, and reduced lung volumes. The loss of lung volume typical of ILD is usually confirmed with restrictive lung function tests and reduced gas-transfer measurements. Often there is a delay in diagnosis whilst patients are treated for lower respiratory tract infections or for pulmonary edema, conditions more prevalent than ILD that commonly form a differential diagnosis until a full clinical assessment including definitive imaging with high-resolution computed tomography (HRCT) is performed (Fig. 9.2).

Idiopathic Pulmonary Fibrosis

Idiopathic pulmonary fibrosis (IPF) is the most common ILD and is the archetypal progressive fibrotic lung disease. IPF is a specific form of chronic fibrosing interstitial lung disease of unknown cause that has an estimated incidence of 5–10 per 100,000 population/year, with the incidence generally accepted to be rising. It is believed that over 500,000 patients are affected by IPF in the USA and Europe. IPF is typically a disease of the elderly, with a mean age of onset of 67 years and is more common in smokers. IPF is characterized by relentless progression of lung fibrosis, impaired lung function, worsening gas exchange, and prominent symptoms of breathlessness and dry cough. Survival of patients with IPF is worse than for many cancers with a median survival of only 3 years from diagnosis.

Whilst population survival in IPF is predictably poor, it is recognized that there is heterogeneity in the clinical course of the disease as well as unpredictable acute worsening or exacerbations of IPF [4]. There appear to be several possible natural histories for patients with IPF which makes accurate prognostication difficult and planning for palliative care and end of life care a particular challenge. The possible natural histories for IPF are summarized in Fig. 9.3. A practical and accurate method to predict the course of the disease and the survival in individual patients has been proposed [5]. In this study, the 1 year mortality of patients with IPF appeared to be predictable, based on modeling retrospective clinical trial data of over 1,000 patients with IPF, using four clinical parameters; age, respiratory hospitalization, forced vital capacity (FVC), expressed as a percentage of the predicted value, and 24 week change in FVC. This approach may facilitate decision- making by patients, carers, and clinical teams, although it clearly needs careful prospective evaluation and validation in other IPF populations before firm recommendations regarding prognostication and guiding clinical management can be made.

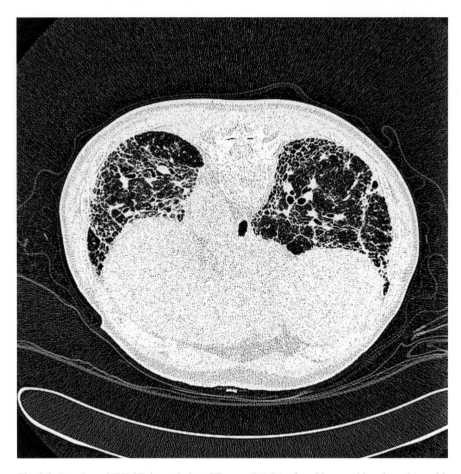

Fig. 9.2 Imaging of IPF. High-resolution CT scan (*HRCT*) of an 82-year-old male patient with advanced IPF. The image, acquired prone, shows evidence of severe basal fibrosis in a typical subpleural distribution, minimal "ground-glass" change, "honeycomb" lung, and evidence of secondary bronchial dilatation. The patient had presented with progressive breathlessness and dry cough. Lung function tests confirmed severe intrapulmonary restriction with low lung volumes and impaired gas transfer. The patient developed worsening respiratory failure and died 18 months from presentation

A number of patients are recognized to have acute worsening of their disease due to identifiable conditions such as pneumonia, pneumothorax, pulmonary embolism, acute coronary syndromes, or cardiac failure. However, it has been estimated that up to 15 % of patients will experience an acute exacerbation of IPF (AE-IPF) each year [6]. These exacerbations are characterized by an acute deterioration (<30 days), with new or worsening breathlessness often accompanied by cough, fever, and flu-like symptoms. Imaging confirms new bilateral ground glass shadowing whilst no other explanation for the exacerbation, including

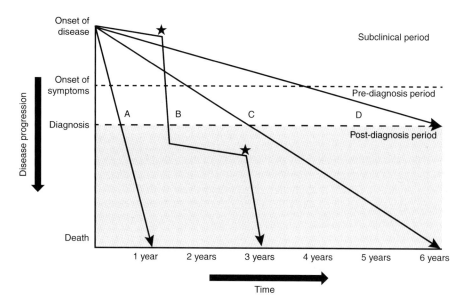

Fig. 9.3 The natural history of IPF (Reproduced with permission from Ley et al. [4]). The variable and unpredictable clinical course of IPF is represented schematically. Following the onset of disease which may be only detectable on high-resolution CT scan or chest radiograph there is a subclinical period. There follows a symptomatic period which is typically present for some time before the diagnosis is secured. The rate of decline may be rapid (*A*), more slowly progressive (*C*) and (*D*) or mixed (*B*) where a relatively indolent deterioration is punctuated with periods of acute decline (*) due to recognized complications such as pneumonia or unexplained AE-IPF. These deteriorations may be fatal or leave the patient with significantly worsened disease

infection, can be identified. Whilst the mechanism of AE-IPF remains unclear and may simply represent an acute acceleration of the fibrotic process underpinning IPF, some authors have speculated that occult viral infection or gastroesophageal reflux disease may play a role [7]. There is no strong evidence on which to base recommendations for the optimal treatment of AE-IPF, although recent guidelines recommend the use of corticosteroids in the majority of these patients [8]. These exacerbations can have a serious impact on both the quality of life and survival of patients with IPF, with up to 50 % of patients dying during an exacerbation [6].

IPF is associated with other diseases that can contribute to worsening symptoms, deterioration and death. It has been recognized that patients with IPF are at significantly increased risk of lung cancer, acute coronary syndromes, and pulmonary embolism. In addition, comorbidities such as pulmonary hypertension and chronic obstructive pulmonary disease (COPD) may contribute to the disease course whilst treatments such as radiotherapy, surgery, and potentially chemotherapy for co-existent lung cancer can precipitate a deterioration or AE-IPF [8, 9].

Intensive Care for Patients with ILD?

Patients with IPF in whom the disease progresses to a stage of respiratory failure may trigger a referral to the intensive care unit (ICU) for consideration of ventilatory support. Available data however show that the outcome for these patients is very poor, mechanical ventilation is mostly futile, and ICU support for these patients is usually not appropriate due to mortality rates of up to 100 % [1]. It is important for the clinical team to be aware of the clinical course of the patient's disease. If a patient has demonstrated the typical inexorable decline in lung function, gas exchange, and symptoms that characterize IPF, it is not appropriate to offer ICU-based organ support. More challenging is the patient with IPF who appears to have an acute deterioration or AE-IPF. In this situation, ICU may be an appropriate setting to perform in a safe and timely fashion the necessary extended investigation to exclude any reversible cause of deterioration in these patients [10]. Patients and their families should be informed about the prognosis, outcome, and overall outlook before making decisions about ventilation and organ support. It is important that all clinicians involved in the management of ILD are aware of the issues relating to the ICU care of these patients and ideally have agreed institutional guidelines which the medical, ICU, and palliative care teams can share [11].

Treatment of IPF

Lee et al. propose a "3 pillars of care" model of for patients with IPF which focuses on (1) disease-centered management, (2) symptom-centered management, and (3) education and self-management [12].

Disease-Centered Management

It is clear that pharmacological treatments aimed at reversing the progressive fibrosis that characterizes IPF have been unsuccessful and often harmful because of significant adverse effects. Traditionally steroids have been used to treat IPF, although no clinical trial data to support their use exist. In the British Thoracic Society ILD Guidelines 2008, a recommendation to use triple therapy with prednisolone, azathioprine, and n-acetylcysteine was made [1]. However, subsequent international guidelines have been unable to recommend the routine use of immunosuppressive drugs and indeed concluded that there is no proven pharmacological therapy for IPF [8]. A recent randomized controlled trial of triple therapy (PANTHER-IPF) was stopped prematurely as patients treated with triple therapy had increased mortality, more serious adverse events, and drug discontinuations, without evidence of benefit. Many other disease-modifying therapies have been tried unsuccessfully and whilst there may be some benefit from the anti-fibrotic drug pirfenidone in selected patients, there is unfortunately no effective drug treatment for progressive IPF. Patients with IPF should be offered participation in well-designed clinical trials with the potential benefits it may bring to both them and other patients in terms of outcomes, symptoms, and quality of life made explicit, although countered by the potential for adverse effects and harm [8].

The use of long-term oxygen therapy (LTOT) has been recommended for patients with IPF who have resting hypoxemia using the same criteria as recommended for patients with COPD [1, 8]. It remains unclear however in the absence of clinical trial data that the survival benefits of LTOT seen in patients with COPD can be extrapolated to patients with IPF.

Lung transplantation is an effective treatment for a minority of patients with IPF. In selected patients, transplantation can dramatically improve the disease trajectory, although timing of referral for assessment remains critical to prevent patients becoming too unwell for consideration of lung transplant or dying on the waiting list [13]. Unfortunately many patients with IPF are elderly and have comorbidities which make them unsuitable for transplantation.

Symptom-Centered Management

The focus on symptom-centered management links with the concept of "best supportive care" as outlined in the British Thoracic Society guidelines and is clearly integral to effective palliative care for a disease which has no proven cure or disease-modifying treatment [1, 8, 12].

An important consideration in being able to proactively identify patients with progressive disease and worsening symptoms is careful monitoring using appropriate clinical evaluation, symptom scores, and quality of life assessments. This approach allows the clinical team to consider therapy choices but also helps patients understand their disease course. The standard objective measures of disease severity and progression are lung function as measured by forced vital capacity (FVC), gas transfer (TLco), oxygenation saturation, and 6 min walk distance. It is widely accepted that a fall in FVC of ≥ 10 % or TLco of ≥ 15 % over a 3–6 month period is indicative of disease progression and a poor outcome. It is clearly important however to ensure that the patient's symptoms are assessed and quantified accurately. Breathlessness is almost universal in patients with IPF, although there is a paucity of data on the clinical utility of assessment tools, most of which were developed for assessment of COPD patients, in this group of patients. Breathlessness has been demonstrated to have a strong correlation with both quality of life and mortality in IPF [14]. Despite its prevalence and prominence, breathlessness has not been the focus of many studies of the natural history or treatment interventions in IPF. The use of a patient-reported measure of breathlessness, Dyspnea-12, has shown promise as a simple, reliable, and valid instrument in patients with ILD [15].

Whilst breathlessness in IPF is principally due to the physiological impact of fibrosis, reduced gas exchange, and ventilation-perfusion mismatching, other factors also influence the patient's perception of breathlessness. In a cross-sectional study of patients with ILD some of whom had IPF, both depression and functional status, as measured by walk distance, were strongly associated with breathlessness [16]. The authors of this study speculated that treatment of depression and programmes of exercise may improve both breathlessness and quality of life.

A dry irritating cough can be a distressing symptom for IPF patients [17]. Cough in IPF is often refractory to anti-tussive therapies and it may be a predictor of progressive disease and mortality [18]. The mechanism of cough in IPF is poorly understood, although it may be due to heightened cough reflex sensitivity [19]. Other co-existent causes of cough, such as gastro-esophageal reflux, upper airway cough syndrome, asthma, and COPD should be considered. There is no IPF-specific tool to assess the severity or impact of a patient's cough, although there appears to be a strong correlation between cough frequency and cough-related quality of life measures [20].

Fatigue in IPF can be a dominant symptom for some patients and can be exacerbated further by muscle deconditioning [17]. Many patients with IPF suffer from anxiety and depression, which can be compounded by the effects of chronic and debilitating symptoms, adverse effects of drug therapies, and fear of disease progression and death [16].

Health-related quality of life (HRQOL) in IPF is now recognized as an important measure to identify changes in the disease process and to quantify the impact of symptoms in individual patients. It is also being increasingly used as an outcome measure in clinical trials. Swigris et al., having recognized the lack of validated HRQOL tools in this disease, interviewed patients in order to identify themes and develop an IPF-specific tool ATAQ-IPF [17, 21]. A modification (SQRQ-I) to the Saint George's Respiratory Questionnaire has been proposed to be reliable for measuring health-related quality of life in patients with IPF [22]. More recently, the King's brief interstitial lung disease questionnaire (K-BILD) has been proposed as a simple tool to assess HRQL in three domains of psychological impact, breathlessness/activities, and chest symptoms [23]. In a pilot study, HRQOL was found to be significantly lower in patients with IPF compared to other ILDs and was also lower in patients with IPF who were prescribed long-term oxygen therapy or immunosuppressant medication. Clearly more studies are needed to assess the longitudinal changes in HRQL using IPF-specific tools and the potential impact of interventions both in research trials and in clinical practice.

Specific Symptom-Centered Treatment

There are a number of approaches that form the foundation of "best supportive care" for patients with IPF. These include smoking cessation, addressing nutrition, treating right heart failure and influenza and pneumococcal vaccination that are likely to improve symptoms and prevent the development of complications. In addition, there are four principal symptoms that should be sought and considered in all patients with IPF.

Breathlessness

A recent systematic review concluded that there were scant data, too much trial heterogeneity to facilitate meta-analysis, and little robust evidence to support the use of specific treatments for the relief of breathlessness in IPF patients [24]. The review suggested that supplemental oxygen, pulmonary rehabilitation, and opioids may be beneficial. BTS guidelines recognize that in the absence of suitable controlled studies of long-term, short burst or ambulatory oxygen therapy in ILD, recommendations are extrapolated from studies in COPD. The guidelines recommend that patients with persistent resting hypoxemia should be considered for palliative oxygen at home delivered by an oxygen concentrator. These individuals may also benefit from ambulatory oxygen if they remain active outside the home. Patients who are not chronically hypoxic but who are breathless, mobile, and exhibit desaturation on exercise should be considered for ambulatory oxygen if improvement in exercise capacity or less breathlessness can be demonstrated by formal ambulatory oxygen assessment. Intermittent supplemental oxygen for periods of 10–20 min at a time and delivered by oxygen cylinder (short burst oxygen therapy) may relieve breathlessness associated with hypoxemia in patients with IPF who do not require an oxygen concentrator or ambulatory oxygen.

A positive impact of pulmonary rehabilitation on breathlessness has been demonstrated with six of seven studies demonstrating an improvement in breathlessness, although only two of these studies were randomized controlled trials of which one showed no improvement [25]. Given the likely benefit in improving breathlessness along with the additional benefits in terms of function and QOL, pulmonary rehabilitation has been recommended for patients with IPF based on the same criteria as for COPD [1, 8]. Specifically tailored rehabilitation for patients with IPF is likely to be beneficial in terms of patient education though no evidence for specific IPF rehabilitation programmes exists and limited resources make delivery of this approach difficult.

Studies of the use of opioids for the relief of breathlessness in IPF are limited. An uncontrolled study of 11 elderly patients with advanced IPF concluded that 2.5 mg of subcutaneous diamorphine and subsequent oral morphine (20–60 mg/day) reduced symptoms of breathlessness with no significant respiratory depression [26]. Guidelines acknowledge that there is no evidence of benefit from nebulized morphine but that oral opiates may be effective in relieving distress from breathlessness in patients with IPF [1]. Pharmacological and non-pharmacological interventions for breathlessness are considered in more detail in Chap. 2.

Cough

There has been limited study of cough as an endpoint of pharmacological intervention. One small study suggested that high-dose oral steroids may improve cough but the routine use of steroids to treat cough in IPF is not recommended because of the potential adverse effects [1]. Oral codeine and stronger opioids as anti-tussives are often used in clinical practice (Chap. 4), although specific evidence to support their use in ILD is lacking. There is some interest in the use of thalidomide in the treatment of IPF-related cough, although clinical data relating to this and novel specific ant-tussive agents are awaited. There is much interest in the potential role of gastro-esophageal reflux disease (GORD) in IPF as this may contribute to the symptom of cough as well as potentially accelerating disease progression. GORD is common in patients with IPF and it is recommended that medical treatment of symptomatic GORD with proton pump inhibitors is considered whilst further studies in this area are concluded [1, 8].

Fatigue and Deconditioning

Fatigue is reported by many IPF patients as a dominant symptom [17], which may not receive the same degree of attention in the clinic as the symptoms of breathless-ness and cough [17]. As is seen in COPD, cardiac and peripheral muscle decondi-tioning can exacerbate fatigue and can lead to a vicious cycle of fatigue, immobility, and deconditioning. Pulmonary rehabilitation has been demonstrated in several small studies to improve walk distance with reduced breathlessness and improved quality of life, presumably through effects on non-pulmonary limitations to exercise in patients with IPF [25]. As in other disease areas, the individual components of a group rehabilitation programme are unlikely to be effective in isolation and it is the multidisciplinary approach to patient assessment, individualized exercise training, nutritional modulation, education and psychosocial counseling that produces benefits for these patients.

It is likely that appropriate use of supplemental oxygen in hypoxemic patients will maximize the efficacy of pulmonary rehabilitation. Furthermore, hypoxemia, including nocturnal hypoxemia, can itself contribute to reduced energy levels and impaired social and physical functioning [27]. Whilst there is a lack of evidence to confirm that treatment with oxygen in this situation is of benefit to patients with ILD, it is important to consider the option of using oxygen and to discuss the practicalities, risks, and benefits with the patient.

Finally, it is important to consider comorbidities such as sleep-disordered breathing as a contributor to fatigue. Studies have suggested that significant obstructive sleep apnea may be present in over two-thirds of IPF patients and should be considered, investigated, and treated [28].

Depression and Anxiety

Many IPF patients experience symptoms of anxiety and depression. A focus group of IPF patients reported sadness, fear, worry, anxiety, and panic, as well as concerns about how the disease impacted on their family and carers. They often reported social isolation and increased dependence on their family [16].

As with the other symptom-centered approaches, there is little evidence for optimal treatment in this specific patient group. An approach to identification and management of anxiety and depression has been proposed and is consistent with our clinical practice [12]:

1. Assess for anxiety and depression using a simple screening tool such as the Hospital Anxiety and Depression Scale (HADS).
2. Use the results of this screening to educate patients and prompt discussions relating to their scores.
3. Consider the role of cognitive behavioral therapy (CBT), advice leaflets, and support groups in treating anxiety or depression.
4. Evaluate for and treat comorbidities contributing to anxiety such as breathlessness, fatigue, and deconditioning.
5. Consider pulmonary rehabilitation.
6. Finally, if not responsive to the above measures, consider specific pharmacological therapy.

Elevated HADS scores are common in IPF. Nearly a quarter of patients had depression in a small cross-sectional study and other studies suggest a correlation with disease duration [29].

The effect of psychoactive medications has not been specifically studied, though it is recommended that serotonin specific reuptake inhibitors (SSRIs) be used in the treatment of depression whilst benzodiazepines or SSRIs can be considered in the treatment of symptoms of anxiety, which has not responded to non-pharmacological approaches [30].

Education and Self-management

From the time of diagnosis patients should be offered individualized but clear and accurate information regarding the diagnosis, treatment options, and prognosis [1]. This includes appropriate written information such as the patient information leaflet supplied with the British Thoracic Society guidelines as well as direction to quality web-based information and materials relating to their disease and its treatment (Table 9.1). A comprehensive IPF education package including information on disease pathophysiology, prognosis and disease trajectory, disease and symptom-centered treatment options including the role of clinical trials has been suggested to allow patients to set realistic goals and to engage in shared decision making. This approach will hopefully allow patients to remain in control of their care, enjoy better quality of life, and prepare for the future [12].

In order that patients, families, and the clinical team can continue to engage in ongoing education and review, regular assessment has been recommended. There will clearly be variability in frequency of follow-up appointments based on patient and disease factors, though 3–6 monthly follow-up is recommended as a minimum for adequate monitoring for disease progression. This frequent contact between the patient and clinical team allows re-assessment of both the patient's and clinician's goals of care.

Table 9.1 Useful resources for education and self-management

Website	Details
http://www.coalitionforpf.org	US-based non-profit organization supporting patients and research into IPF
http://www.pulmonaryfibrosis.org.uk	UK-based patient education and support organization
http://www.lunguk.org	British Lung Foundation patient support charity with UK wide local patient/carer groups
http://www.pulmonary-fibrosis.net	European wide research and clinical trial consortium
http://pulmonaryfibrosis.org	US-based non-profit organization supporting patients and research into IPF
http://www.brit-thoracic.org.uk	British Thoracic Society Guidelines and supporting patient information
http://www.european-lung-foundation.org	European Respiratory Society supported patient/professional resource
http://www.pilotforipf.org	US-based continuing medical education programme for health professionals

The structure of clinical services shows variability within countries as well as internationally. There is recognition that, in view of the diagnostic challenges involved, specialist regional ILD multidisciplinary teams are needed to support clinicians and patients in securing an accurate diagnosis and thus prognosis, often in a "shared care" approach with the local clinicians. Guidelines and emerging standards of care for ILD recognize the role of a multidisciplinary team in supporting the ILD patient that should include a nurse specialist and access to a specialist palliative care team. However, a recent UK survey showed that there was significant variation in practice and access to these services. Of 120 UK centers responding, only 57 % ran an ILD clinic and only 47 % had an ILD multidisciplinary team. Whilst the majority of centers had access to ambulatory oxygen services, pulmonary rehabilitation and specialist palliative care teams only a quarter had an ILD nurse specialist [31].

An important aspect of patient education and self-management is advance care planning (Chap. 14). It is important that issues relating to advance care planning are considered and discussed, ideally at a non-critical time, when death is not imminent – anticipating rather than reacting to the unpredictable and progressive nature of IPF.

In a recent retrospective survey of the palliative care needs of IPF patients, 17 of 45 patients had specialist palliative care team involvement [32]. Nearly all patients (42 of 45) experienced breathlessness in their last year of life. Additional symptoms included cough, fatigue, depression, anxiety, and chest pain. All patients given opioids (22 of 45) or benzodiazepines (8 of 45) showed an improvement in symptoms. Non-pharmacological treatments were rarely used. Few patients had had their preferred place of care (8 of 45) or preferred place of death (6 of 45) documented. The authors concluded that non-pharmacological interventions were seldom used and that documentation of preferred place of care and preferred place of death was poor.

In order to address patient's wishes that they "wanted assurance that their symptoms would be controlled, that their passing would be peaceful and that the dying process would occur on their terms," clearer guidance and education relating to end of life care in ILD is required [17].

Integrating Palliative Care into an ILD Service

Since there is no current treatment that can effectively prevent disease progression in IPF, it is important that palliative care starts is incorporated into the management of these patients from the time of diagnosis. Various models of palliative care have been proposed. A model of palliative care that starts when curative/restorative care ends is clearly not appropriate in ILD. The model best suited to management of IPF is that involving individualized, integrated palliative care [30]. In this model, the patient receives palliative care from the outset of symptoms and concurrently with disease-centered management. The intensity of palliative care is adjusted to reflect the needs of patients and their carers, and often increases towards the end of life.

In recognizing the often scant evidence base supporting palliative care approaches to the management of these patients, there is clearly a need for further high-quality clinical trials. These should focus on outcomes relevant to patients that look not only at new disease-centered treatments but also at symptom-centered approaches. Current international ILD guidelines offer the clinical team some advice on palliative care approaches, certainly more than their previous iterations, but perhaps not surprisingly there is often more attention given to the increasing list of non-effective disease-modifying approaches to IPF [1, 8].

The complexity of ILD requires a close working relationship between patients and their healthcare professionals as well as between members of the clinical team who need to deliver both general and specialist palliative care from the outset of the patient's journey. It is recommended that palliative care specialists form part of the ILD multidisciplinary team.

A "top ten points approach" to palliative care of ILD is suggested:

1. Use a multidisciplinary approach to secure the correct diagnosis.
2. Ensure the patient and their family have access to high-quality information about their disease and access to appropriate support both in the clinic and at home.
3. Offer the patient access to clinical trials looking at both disease-centered and symptom-centered outcomes.
4. Monitor the patient closely for symptoms and evidence of deterioration to inform the need for intervention and to obtain prognostic information, referring patients early for consideration of lung transplantation where appropriate, as this is the only current treatment with significant prognostic advantage.
5. Ensure avoidance, dose reduction, or withdrawal of therapy that has no benefit and may do harm.
6. Ensure all patients have access to smoking cessation support, pulmonary rehabilitation, and oxygen services.
7. Actively enquire about and measure breathlessness, cough, fatigue, anxiety, and depression.

8. Accept the limited clinical data in treating symptoms of IPF but treat actively using a trials of treatment in individual patients.
9. Consider the use of opioids and benzodiazepines for the relief of breathlessness and strategies such as cognitive behavioral therapy (CBT) to treat anxiety.
10. Share decision making with the patient and family, and actively discuss and end of life issues.

References

1. Wells AU, Hirani N. British Thoracic Society – interstitial lung disease guideline. Thorax. 2008;63 Suppl 5:1–58.
2. Flaherty KR, King TE, Raghu G, et al. Idiopathic interstitial pneumonia. Am J Respir Crit Care Med. 2004;170:904–10.
3. American Thoracic Society/European Respiratory Society international multidisciplinary consensus classification of the idiopathic interstitial pneumonias. Am J Respir Crit Care Med. 2002;165:277–304.
4. Ley B, Collard HR, King TE. Clinical course and prediction of survival in idiopathic pulmonary fibrosis. Am J Respir Crit Care Med. 2011;183:431–40.
5. du Bois RM, Weycker D, Albera C, et al. Ascertainment of individual risk of mortality for patients with idiopathic pulmonary fibrosis. Am J Respir Crit Care Med. 2011;184:459–66.
6. Song JW, Hong SB, Lim CM, et al. Acute exacerbation of idiopathic pulmonary fibrosis: incidence, risk factors and outcome. Eur Respir J. 2011;37(2):356–63.
7. Collard HR, Moore BB, Flaherty KR, et al. Acute exacerbations of idiopathic pulmonary fibrosis. Am J Respir Crit Care Med. 2007;176:636–43.
8. Raghu G, Collard HR, Egan JJ, et al. An official ATS/ERS/JRS/ALAT statement: idiopathic pulmonary fibrosis: evidence-based guidelines for diagnosis and management. Am J Respir Crit Care Med. 2011;183:788–824.
9. Raghu G, Nyberg F, Morgan G. The epidemiology of interstitial lung disease and its association with lung cancer. Br J Cancer. 2004;91 Suppl 2:S3–10.
10. Papiris SA, Manali ED, Kolilekas L, et al. Clinical review: idiopathic pulmonary fibrosis acute exacerbations – unravelling Ariadne's thread. Crit Care. 2010;14:246–56.
11. Mallick S. Outcome of patients with idiopathic pulmonary fibrosis ventilated in intensive care unit. Respir Med. 2008;102:1355–9.
12. Lee JS, McLaughlin S, Collard HR. Comprehensive care of the patient with idiopathic pulmonary fibrosis. Curr Opin Pulm Med. 2011;17:348–54.
13. Mackay LS, Anderson RL, Parry G, et al. Pulmonary fibrosis: rate of disease progression as a trigger for referral for lung transplantation. Thorax. 2007;62:1069–73.
14. Swigris JJ, Kuschner WG, Jacobs SS, et al. Health-related quality of life in patients with idiopathic pulmonary fibrosis: a systematic review. Thorax. 2005;60:588–94.
15. Yorke J, Swigris JJ, Russell AM, et al. Dyspnoea-12 is a valid and reliable measure of breathlessness in patients with ILD. Chest. 2010;139:159–64.
16. Ryerson CJ, Berkeley J, Carrieri-Kohlman VL, et al. Depression and functional status are strongly associated with dyspnea in interstitial lung disease. Chest. 2011;139:609–16.
17. Swigris JJ, Stewart AL, Gould MK, et al. Patients' perspectives on how idiopathic pulmonary fibrosis affects the quality of their lives. Health Qual Life Outcomes. 2005;3:61–70.
18. Ryerson CJ, Abbritti M, Ley B, et al. Cough predicts prognosis in idiopathic pulmonary fibrosis. Respirology. 2011;16:969–75.
19. Hope-Gill BDM, Hilldrup S, Davies C, et al. A study of the cough reflex in idiopathic pulmonary fibrosis. Am J Respir Crit Care Med. 2003;168:995–1002.

20. Key AL, Holt K, Hamilton A, et al. Objective cough frequency in idiopathic pulmonary fibrosis. Cough. 2010;6:4.
21. Swigris JJ, Wilson SR, Green KE, et al. Development of the ATAQ-IPF: a tool to assess quality of life in IPF. Health Qual Life Outcomes. 2010;8:77.
22. Yorke J, Jones PW, Swigris JJ. Development and validity testing of an IPF-specific version of the St George's Respiratory Questionnaire. Thorax. 2010;65:921–6.
23. Patel AS, Siegert R, Brignall K, et al. T he assessment of health-related quality of life in interstitial lung disease with the King's brief interstitial lung disease questionnaire (K-BILD). Thorax. 2011;66 Suppl 4:A61.
24. Ryerson CJ, Donesky D, Pantilat SZ, et al. Dyspnea in idiopathic pulmonary fibrosis: a systematic review. J Pain Symptom Manage. 2012;43:771–82.
25. Ryerson CJ, Garvey C, Collard HR. Pulmonary rehabilitation for interstitial lung disease. Chest. 2010;138:240–1.
26. Allen S, Raut S, Woollard J, et al. Low dose diamorphine reduces breathlessness without causing a fall in oxygen saturation in elderly patients with end-stage idiopathic pulmonary fibrosis. Palliat Med. 2005;19:128–30.
27. Clark M, Cooper B, Singh S, et al. A survey of nocturnal hypoxaemia and health-related quality of life in patients with cryptogenic fibrosing alveolitis. Thorax. 2001;56:482–6.
28. Lancaster LH, Mason WR, Parnell JA, et al. Obstructive sleep apnea is common in idiopathic pulmonary fibrosis. Chest. 2009;136:772–8.
29. Spruit MA, Janssen DJA, Franssen FME, et al. Rehabilitation and palliative care in lung fibrosis. Respirology. 2009;14:781–7.
30. Lanken PN, Terry PB, Delisser HM, et al. An official American Thoracic Society clinical policy statement: palliative care for patients with respiratory diseases and critical illnesses. Am J Respir Crit Care Med. 2008;177:912–27.
31. Dempsey OJ, Welham S, Hirani N. BTS national interstitial lung diseases (ILD) survey 2010–2011. Thorax. 2011;66 Suppl 4:A102.
32. Bajwah S, Higginson IJ, Ross JR. Specialist palliative care is more than drugs: a retrospective study of ILD patients. Lung. 2012;190:215–20.

Chapter 10
Cystic Fibrosis

Stephen J. Bourke and Rachel Quibell

Abstract Although the prognosis of patients with cystic fibrosis continues to improve, many still die in early adulthood of respiratory failure. As the disease progresses patients have a high level of complex symptoms and a high burden of treatment. Palliative care is intertwined with potential lung transplantation, but not all patients are suitable for transplantation and the shortage of donor organs means that up to 40 % of patients on a transplant waiting list die before donor organs become available. Disease-modifying therapies, supportive care, emergency care, and palliative care all run in parallel for these patients. Palliative care is a key component of a comprehensive adult cystic fibrosis service, and this is often organized in an integrated model of care with specialist palliative care clinicians forming part of the multidisciplinary CF team and working collaboratively with the CF team.

Keywords Cystic fibrosis • Lung transplantation • Palliative care • Transplant trajectory • Multidisciplinary team

Although the prognosis of patients with cystic fibrosis (CF) continues to improve, many still die in early adulthood. National registries show that in 2009 there were 141 deaths from CF in the UK and 440 in the USA [1, 2]. The age range for deaths in the UK was from 9 to 82 years with a median of 27 years (Fig. 10.1). Nowadays very few deaths occur in childhood, the majority occur in early adulthood, and an increasing number occur in middle to older age. This reflects the improved prognosis

S.J. Bourke, M.D., FRCP, FRCPI, DCH (✉)
Department of Respiratory Medicine, Royal Victoria Infirmary,
Queen Victoria Road, Newcastle upon Tyne NE1 4LP, UK
e-mail: Stephen.Bourke@nuth.nhs.uk

R. Quibell, M.B.B.S., FRCP
Department of Palliative Medicine, Royal Victoria Infirmary,
Newcastle upon Tyne, UK

S.J. Bourke, E.T. Peel (eds.), *Integrated Palliative Care of Respiratory Disease*,
DOI 10.1007/978-1-4471-2230-2_10, © Springer-Verlag London 2013

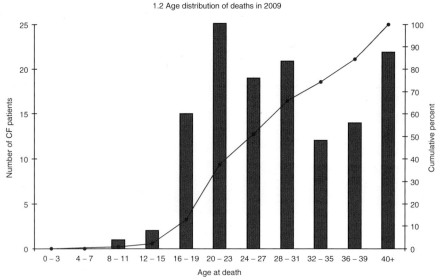

There were 141 recorded deaths in 2009. The median age at death was 27 years (min = 9 Years; max = 82 years)

Fig. 10.1 Age distribution of deaths from cystic fibrosis in the UK 2009. Nowadays very few deaths occur in childhood, the majority occur in early adulthood, and an increasing number occur in middle to older age (Reproduced with permission from the Cystic Fibrosis Trust annual data report [1])

of the disease with intensive treatment in specialist centers and also the recognition of a spectrum of severity of the disease which includes some milder cases. The vast majority of deaths are due to respiratory failure. Palliative care of patients with CF is often undertaken by CF teams rather than palliative care teams because of the specialist nature of the disease and the potential role of lung transplantation, which is paradoxically intertwined with palliative care. The transition from disease-modifying treatments to palliative care is particularly complex. Palliative care is a crucial component of a comprehensive adult CF service [3].

Overview of Cystic Fibrosis

CF is an autosomal recessive disease caused by mutations of a gene on chromosome 7 that encodes for a protein named cystic fibrosis transmembrane conductance regulator (CFTR), which functions as a chloride channel in the apical membrane of epithelial cells [4]. Reduced chloride conductance results in viscid secretions and organ damage in the respiratory, gastrointestinal, hepatobiliary, and reproductive tracts. It affects about 1 in 2,500 births in the UK, and about 1 in 25 of the population is a carrier of the disease.

More than 1,800 mutations of the CF gene have been identified and this partly explains the wide spectrum of severity of the disease, although other factors such as environmental factors and modifier genes affecting the inflammatory response are also important. The most common mutation, traditionally known as ΔF508 (F508del), results in the loss of phenylalanine at position 508 of the protein. This causes misfolding of the mutant CFTR, which is then degraded such that no CFTR reaches the cell membrane. In certain mutations, the mutant CFTR retains some function and this may be associated with less severe disease. Some rare patients have non-classic CF in which they have two mutations of the gene, abnormal sweat chloride, some manifestations of the disease (such as male infertility, pancreatitis, and nasal polyps) but little or no lung disease. There is a spectrum of severity and the treatment regimen is adjusted according to the type, severity, stage, and complications of the disease.

The CF gene has been cloned and given to patients using liposomes or inactivated viruses as gene transfer agents. Expression of the gene has been confirmed by measuring transepithelial potential difference and trials are in progress to assess whether gene therapy can improve clinical outcomes. Substantial progress is being made in treatments that address the molecular biology processes of CFTR transcription from DNA, trafficking through the cell and activation and regulation at the cell membrane [4]. Some treatments are targeted at specific mutations. Thus a small molecule, named Ataluren® (PTC Therapeutics), induces ribosomes to read through premature termination codons during mRNA translation of certain mutations (such as G542X and W1282X). Ivacaftor® (Vx770; Vertex Pharmaceuticals) is a CFTR potentiator that improves CFTR function in patients with the G551D mutation. These new treatments are likely to improve the outcome for patients now being born with CF, but are likely to be of less benefit to those who already have advanced lung disease.

In the bronchial mucosa, reduced chloride secretion and increased sodium reabsorption result in secretions of abnormal viscosity with reduced water content of the airway surface liquid and disrupted mucociliary clearance. This predisposes to chronic infection with associated inflammation progressing to bronchiectasis, respiratory failure, and death. Initially infection is often with *Staphylococcus aureus*. Subsequently, *Pseudomonas aeruginosa* becomes the dominant pathogen. Different strains of pseudomonas can be identified and they vary in their virulence and transmissibility. *Burkholderia cepacia* complex is a group of Gram-negative bacteria which have a high level of antibiotic resistance. Patients with CF are vulnerable to these bacteria and infection can spread from patient to patient. The most virulent strains are *B cenocepacia* and *B multivorans*. Non-tuberculous mycobacteria (such as *Mycobacterium abscessus*) can also infect the lungs in CF and are difficult to treat. Patients are segregated according to their infections when attending hospital and contact between patients is discouraged.

In the pancreas, plugging and obstruction of ductules causes progressive destruction of the gland. Pancreatic enzymes (such as lipase) fail to reach the small intestine and this results in malabsorption of fats with steatorrhea and weight loss. Approximately 40 % of adults develop diabetes from destruction of the endocrine pancreas. Lack of pancreatic enzymes with viscid intestinal secretions and reduced motility can result in distal intestinal obstruction, which is usually treated by intestinal lavage and osmotic agents (such as Gastrografin®). Men with CF are nearly always infertile because of obstruction of the vas deferens but can achieve biological parenthood by sperm aspiration from the testes with in vitro fertilization. Women with CF have essentially normal fertility and many undertake pregnancy and motherhood, but may not survive to see the child reach adulthood.

The key elements of treatment are clearance of bronchial secretions by physiotherapy, treatment of pulmonary infection by antibiotics, and correction of nutritional defects by pancreatic enzyme supplements and dietary support [5]. Patients are typically given flucloxacillin continuously to prevent or suppress *Staphylococcus aureus* infection. When Pseudomonas is first isolated, attempts are made to eradicate it by prolonged courses of oral ciprofloxacin and nebulized colistin or tobramycin. When pseudomonas infection becomes established, long-term nebulized antibiotics are used to suppress infection. Exacerbations are treated by combinations of intravenous antibiotics (such as ceftazidime or meropenem with tobramycin or colistin). Treatment is facilitated by use of indwelling central venous access devices and many patients self-administer antibiotics intravenously at home (Fig. 10.2). As the disease progresses, the frequency of antibiotics increases. Even in late stage disease intravenous antibiotics are effective in improving the level of symptoms. Malabsorption is controlled by use of pancreatic enzymes with food. As the chest disease progresses, patients have difficulty in maintaining their energy requirements because of decreased appetite and the increased energy expenditure associated with chronic lung infection. Dietary supplements are used when anorexia limits intake and supplemental feeding is often given overnight via a gastrostomy tube. Mucolytic agents, such as nebulized 7 % saline or deoxyribonuclease (DNase), aid clearance of airway secretions. Lung transplantation is the main treatment for patients with end-stage lung disease but lack of donor organs limits this treatment. Overall survival rates post-transplantation are approximately 80 % at 1 year, 60 % at 5 years, and 50 % at 10 years [6]. Palliative care is paradoxically intertwined with high-intensity treatments including lung transplantation and many patients who die will be on a transplant waiting list at the time of death.

Predicting the Prognosis

Patients with CF live their lives in the knowledge of having a chronic life-limiting disease. They show remarkable resilience in the face of the disease: "I do not sit around worrying about when I am going to die. I will worry about the future when it arrives. I think about it but do not walk around clutching my funeral arrangements" [7]. At present the median survival is about 38 years but it is predicted to be at least 50 years for children now being born with the disease [8]. In most patients, there is a gradual, generally predictable progression of lung disease that allows a planned approach to both lung transplantation and palliative care. However, patients can suffer an acute crisis from complications such as massive hemoptysis,

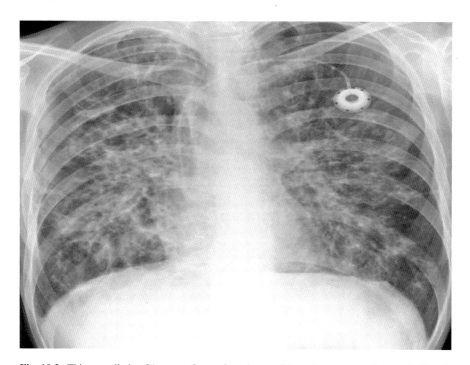

Fig. 10.2 This man died at 21 years of age of respiratory failure from progressive cystic fibrosis lung disease. Two years previously he had been deemed unsuitable for lung transplantation because of *Burkholderia cenocepacia* infection. He had a prolonged phase of palliative care of advanced disease during which he had supplemental gastrostomy feeding, intensive physiotherapy, and frequent courses of intravenous antibiotics. He also attended a specialist palliative care symptom-control clinic, but he did not find a hospice day care facility helpful. His chest radiograph shows severe diffuse bronchiectasis and a central venous access system in the left subclavian vein. After several exacerbations he deteriorated into terminal stage disease and died at home with end of life care from the community palliative care team

pneumothorax, or a severe acute exacerbation. Lung transplantation is generally considered at a stage where the forced expiratory volume in one second (FEV1) has fallen to below 30 % of the predicted value. Some studies suggest that this indicates an approximately 50 % risk of dying within 2 years [9]. Additional factors such as the rate of decline, frequency of exacerbations, development of hypoxia and hypercapnia, and occurrence of complications are also important in predicting a poor prognosis. However, the advanced stage of the disease is often a prolonged phase over many years, and intensive treatment with frequent courses of intravenous antibiotics, mucolytic agents, physiotherapy, and nutritional support can improve the survival and quality of life for these patients [10]. Some patients are unsuitable for transplantation because of resistant infections (such as *Burkholderia cenocepacia*, *Mycobacterium abscessus*), poor nutritional status, or additional systemic disease (such as renal disease). Some patients do not wish to undergo transplantation because they fear high-risk intensive treatments. The shortage of donor organs means that up to 40 % of patients considered suitable for transplantation die before donor lungs become available [11].

As with many chronic lung diseases, there is often a prolonged phase of advanced disease requiring symptom control and palliative supportive care followed by a short terminal phase. Precise prediction of the likely time of death is often not possible or helpful, and many of these patients have already survived beyond the life expectancy given to them in childhood. Often it is better to acknowledge that when the disease is progressing and transplantation is not feasible the aim of treatment is to keep patients "as well as possible for as long as possible and to focus on keeping them comfortable when the time comes." This equates to a goal of optimizing the quality of life and ensuring a peaceful, dignified natural death. Many will have specific aims which they want to achieve within their limited life expectancy, such as bringing-up a young child. The classic disease trajectory of cancer patients, with a gradual switch from active treatments to palliation over a relatively short time period, does not apply to patients with CF where palliative care principles are applicable at all stages of the disease, run in parallel with disease-modifying treatments and are still appropriate for patients who ultimately undergo a rescue lung transplant. In a cancer trajectory, care will often transfer from the medical team to the palliative care team, whereas in the chronic illness trajectory integration of palliative care into the multidisciplinary management of the disease is often more appropriate.

Symptom Control in Advanced Disease

In advanced CF, patients often have a range of complex problems. Symptoms can be both physical and psychological. The dominant physical symptoms are cough, sputum, wheeze, chest tightness, breathlessness, pain, fever, and fatigue [12, 13]. The emotional impact of these symptoms is high, and when combined with a realization that the prognosis is poor, results in frustration, anger, sadness, irritability, worry, and difficulty sleeping. A study of self-reported symptom burden revealed that patients had a median of ten different symptoms [13]. These symptoms and the emotional response impact on activities with more time spent sitting or lying, a reduction in usual activities, and missing work. Pain is a common symptom at all stages of CF but becomes more prominent as the disease progresses. Surveys show that 84 % of patients with advanced CF have pain: 65 % have chest pain, 55 % headaches, 19 % back pain, and 19 % abdominal pain [14]. The majority of chest and back pain is of musculoskeletal origin related to use of accessory muscles of respiration, coughing, postural abnormalities, or osteoporosis. Several studies suggest that the problems of chronic pain in CF are not adequately addressed with a lack of use of analgesic medication or other treatment strategies for pain [14, 15]. When assessing patients with CF in addition to focusing on key elements of the disease such as lung function, oxygenation, nutritional status, and control of infection, it may also be helpful to use symptom check lists to identify the symptom burden, the emotional impact of these symptoms, and the impact these symptoms are having on activities and quality of life [12, 13]. Symptom control requires detailed assessment and a multifaceted approach. Specific treatments directed against the disease, such as a course of intravenous antibiotics, result in improvements in quality of life and in multiple domains of the chronic disease questionnaire [12]. Some symptoms, such as hemoptysis, may require a specific intervention such as bronchial artery embolization. Other specific interventions targeting specific symptoms include analgesia for pain, sputum clearance physiotherapy for cough and secretions, mucolytics for sputum retention, and anti-emetics for nausea and vomiting. Management of psychological symptoms should be part of a holistic approach.

It is also advisable to continually assess the burden of treatment. With disease progression there is often a need to intensify treatments but this may impair quality of life further. An ever increasing treatment regimen may not be effective as patients may have difficulty coping with it. A survey of 204 patients found a mean reported time spent on treatment of 108 min each day, even though less than half these patients had performed their recommended physiotherapy airway clearance techniques [16].

Increasingly health-related quality of life is used in the clinical assessment of patients with CF and as an outcome measure in clinical trials [17]. This describes the state of well-being in terms of the ability to perform everyday activities and reflects physical, psychological, and social well-being as well as satisfaction with levels of functioning, control of disease, and treatment-related symptoms. As in other chronic lung diseases, lung function measurements are poor predictors of the degree of disability. Cognitive and behavioral factors are important in the patient's perception of their health and in the way they cope with and adapt to the disease. Cognitive behavioral therapy is a treatment for emotional and adjustment problems. It addresses unhelpful thinking and worrying and promotes understanding of how thoughts, mood, behavior, and physical symptoms interact. It is effective in reducing anxiety and depression scores in patients with CF [18]. The CF quality of life questionnaire is a measurement of 52 items across nine domains: physical functioning, social functioning, treatment issues, chest symptoms, emotional functioning, concerns for the future, interpersonal relationships, body image, and carer concerns [17]. It can be used to complement clinical measures of disease status and to identify issues requiring further specific interventions.

There may be an important role for specialist palliative services in symptom control at a much earlier stage of the disease than is currently commonly the case. Paradoxically the time when lung transplantation is being considered as an option may also be a useful point to focus on palliative care, either as a specific approach by the CF multidisciplinary team or by a palliative care physician or nurse specialist. Introduction to specialist palliative care before there is a crisis may be helpful in allaying fears and misconceptions.

Dying with Cystic Fibrosis

The circumstances of death differ from patient to patient [3]. Most have a gradual progressive deterioration that allows a planned approach to palliative care. Some suffer a sudden crisis due to a major hemoptysis, pneumothorax, or a severe exacerbation such that there is an abrupt change from being reasonably well to being terminally ill. Some die on a transplant waiting list when there is an attitude of "fighting on" followed by "unfulfilled hope." Some patients die after transplantation from transplant complications or from rejection of the donor lungs.

Typically the dying phase starts with a patient presenting with a further exacerbation with an increase in cough, sputum, and breathlessness [3, 19–21]. Often the patient has recovered from many such exacerbations previously. The patient, family, and CF team initially expect a response to treatment and it may be only after several days of treatment that it becomes apparent that the patient is deteriorating. There is then a transition from the phase of management of chronic advanced disease to the dying phase and terminal care. Patients dying of CF usually have a high level of complex symptoms requiring palliation. The dominant symptom is breathlessness and this is frequently linked to anxiety and fear in a vicious cycle. It is often accompanied by difficulty in expectorating sputum with retained secretions, chest tightness, and pain [3].

Breathlessness is usually alleviated by a combination of drug treatments, such as midazolam and opioids, and general measures such as oxygen, nursing in an upright position, use of a cool air fan, breathing control methods, reassurance and distraction techniques to encourage the patient to focus on issues other than the sensation of breathing. Cognitive behavioral therapy is sometimes useful in helping to break the vicious cycle of breathlessness, anxiety, and fear [18]. This involves recognition that it is not just the impact of a physical symptom but the patient's perception and response to the symptom that may be important. There is often a particular role for the physiotherapist in using breathing control techniques to relieve breathlessness and airway clearance techniques to relieve sputum retention. Hyoscine may be helpful in reducing secretions in the final hours of life. Other common symptoms are cough, hemoptysis, headache, and abdominal pain but these are often masked by the dominance of breathlessness as the main symptom. A particularly difficult symptom to alleviate is a sensation of general malaise, often described as "feeling awful." This is probably due to a combination of lung sepsis, hypoxia, and terminal debility of the dying phase.

Some patients may be receiving non-invasive ventilation to relieve symptoms of hypercapnic respiratory failure [22]. This has been shown to improve symptoms and quality of life in advanced stage disease, but it may no longer be appropriate in the dying phase when the focus is on relieving distress as life peacefully comes to a natural end, rather than on prolonging dying. Similarly endotracheal ventilation on an intensive care unit is usually avoided, although it may be appropriate in the initial management of an acute crisis related to a potentially reversible cause such as pneumothorax or massive hemoptysis [23]. End of life care is particularly complex when the patient is on a transplant waiting list [24]. Some patients with advanced respiratory failure remain suitable for transplantation and some who die have had a transplant "call out" within a week of their death but not received a transplant as the donor organs proved unsuitable [3]. Although full palliative symptom-relieving treatments are given, it can be difficult, and perhaps inappropriate, to address some end of life issues such as "saying goodbye" when a patient is awaiting transplantation as the focus is on "fighting on" in the hope of rescue transplantation. Stopping some treatments during the final stages of the disease requires careful consideration.

Antibiotics and mucolytic drugs are often continued for symptom relief. Many patients still find physiotherapy helpful with the techniques adapted for relief of breathlessness, cough, and retained secretions. Patients also fear being abandoned by the CF team and it may be important for dieticians, nurses, and physiotherapists to continue to visit to provide support. It is usual for members of the team to attend the funeral and to be available to meet the family during the bereavement phase.

Most end of life care is delivered by adult CF teams using the Liverpool care pathway for the dying, with support from specialist palliative care teams. At present, most CF deaths occur in hospital rather than at home or in a hospice [3, 19–21]. Even patients who have indicated in advance that they would wish to be at home when dying often chose to be in hospital when the terminal phase occurs. This may be because of the high level of complex symptoms and because of the typical pattern of the final illness presenting initially with a potentially reversible crisis. Specialist palliative care teams may have a particular role in involving community palliative care services so as to allow patients to return home to die if that is their wish and in some cases transfer to a hospice may be appropriate. It is increasingly common for patients dying from CF to have their own children, or siblings who may also have CF, visiting during the terminal illness and their needs must also be met [3].

Detailed interviews with patients, families, and CF teams indicate that there are unmet needs in palliative care, and the patients and families look to the CF team to initiate end of life discussions [25]. They may be reluctant to have care transferred to a different team or to a hospice setting, but usually welcome the input of specialists in palliative care as part of the multidisciplinary CF team. Often a specialist palliative care consultation will start by focusing on symptoms and then move on to explore the patient's fears, expectations, and wishes, at a time and pace which suits the individual patient.

It is good practice for members of the CF and palliative care teams to discuss and reflect on how the patient's death was managed. This can be a valuable learning opportunity for both teams. CF teams who have not had training or experience of palliative care may have difficulty in coping with end-stage CF. They may experience a sense of failure in the face of the disease. Unwittingly they may distance themselves from the dying patient with a concept that "nothing more can be done." This may particularly be the case in pediatrics where teams are nowadays unlikely to have much experience of the death of CF patients. However, most adult CF teams now recognize palliative care as a key component of a comprehensive service [26]. Although the death of young adults from CF is inherently sad and distressing, it is a privilege, and professionally fulfilling, to manage their care in the palliative stages of the disease.

Organization of Palliative and End of Life Care

The organization of palliative care services for patients with CF needs to be flexible. Patients follow their own particular disease pathway and have their own needs and wishes. In some cases, it may be appropriate to have most care transferred to a hospice or community palliative team. In many cases, it is more appropriate to integrate palliative care into the CF multidisciplinary team. Adult CF teams need to develop links with specialist palliative care services in order to develop an integrated service. Palliative physicians and nurses may then form part of the wider CF team and attend team meetings to support staff in the care of these patients and to identify patients who would benefit from additional specialist palliative care input. This allows all members of the CF team to develop the skills, knowledge, and ethos of palliation and it also allows the palliative care team to understand the problems and complexity of CF care.

There are two main phases to palliative care of CF: a phase of management of advanced disease which is often prolonged, and a phase of terminal care of the dying patient which is often short. Patients and their families look to CF teams to initiate discussions about end of life issues and generally indicate that such discussions currently occur too late [25]. The point at which the role and limitations of lung transplantation are being considered may also be a useful time to focus specifically on palliative care. At this stage the CF team is focused on the decline in lung function, the options for intensifying treatment and the potential role of lung transplantation. These discussions provide an opportunity for considering the poor prognosis, the risk of dying, the burden and impact of symptoms, the role of palliative care, and the patient's plans and wishes. The patient may benefit from a specialist palliative care consultation at this stage. This introduces patients to the palliative care team and in some cases they may benefit from a specific symptom-control approach. The end of life phase of the disease often arises when the patient has presented with a further exacerbation which then fails to respond to treatment and the focus of care transitions to terminal care which is often delivered by the CF team using the Liverpool care pathway for the dying. Involvement of specialist palliative care services at this stage can bring additional expertise in addressing several issues, such as control of complex symptoms, communication with the patient and family, and involvement of community services to facilitate care and death at home if the patient wishes this, with bereavement support.

References

1. Cystic Fibrosis Trust. UK CF registry annual data report 2009. Bromley: Cystic Fibrosis Trust; 2009. www.cftrust.org.uk/CF_Registry_summary.pdf. Accessed on 2012.
2. Cystic Fibrosis Foundation. Patient registry annual data report 2009. Bethesda: Cystic Fibrosis Foundation; 2009. www.cff.org/LivingWithCF/CareCenterNetwork/PatientRegistry/. Accessed on 2012.
3. Bourke SJ, Doe SJ, Gascoigne AD, et al. An integrated model of provision of palliative care to patients with cystic fibrosis. Palliat Med. 2009;23:512–7.
4. Rogan MP, Stoltz DA, Hornick DB. Cystic fibrosis transmembrane conductance regulator intracellular processing, trafficking, and opportunities for mutation-specific treatment. Chest. 2011;139:1480–90.

5. Cohen-Cymberknoh M, Shoseyov D, Kerem E. Managing cystic fibrosis: strategies that increase life expectancy and improve quality of life. Am J Respir Crit Care Med. 2011;183: 1463–71.
6. Meachery G, DeSoyza A, Nicholson A, et al. Outcomes of lung transplantation for cystic fibrosis in a large UK cohort. Thorax. 2008;63:725–31.
7. Wicks E. A patient's journey: cystic fibrosis. BMJ. 2007;334:1270–1.
8. Dodge JA, Lewis PA, Stanton M, Wilsher J. Cystic fibrosis mortality and survival in the UK: 1947-2003. Eur Respir J. 2007;29:522–6.
9. Kerem E, Reisman J, Corey M, Canny GJ, Levison H. Prediction of mortality in patient's with cystic fibrosis. N Engl J Med. 1992;326:1187–91.
10. George PM, Banya W, Pareek N, et al. Improved survival at low lung function in cystic fibrosis: cohort study from 1990 to 2007. BMJ. 2011;342:586–7.
11. Mayer-Hamblett N, Rosenfield M, Emerson J, Goss CH, Aitken ML. Developing cystic fibrosis lung transplant referral criteria using predictors of 2-year mortality. Am J Respir Crit Care Med. 2002;166:1550–5.
12. Goss CH, Edwards TC, Ramsey BW, Aitken ML, Patrick DL. Patient-reported respiratory symptoms in cystic fibrosis. J Cyst Fibros. 2009;8:245–52.
13. Sawicki GS, Sellers DE, Robinson WM. Self-reported physical and psychological symptom burden in adults with cystic fibrosis. J Pain Symptom Manage. 2008;35:372–80.
14. Ravilly S, Robinson W, Suresh S, Wohl ME, Berde CB. Chronic pain in cystic fibrosis. Pediatrics. 1996;98:741–7.
15. Stenekes SJ, Hughes A, Gregoire MC, Frager G, Robinson WM, McGrath PJ. Frequency and self-management of pain, dyspnea and cough in cystic fibrosis. J Pain Symptom Manage. 2009;38:837–48.
16. Sawicki GS, Sellers DE, Robinson WM. High treatment burden in adults with cystic fibrosis: challenges to disease self-management. J Cyst Fibros. 2009;8:91–6.
17. Gee L, Abbott J, Conway SP, Etherington C, Webb AK. Development of a disease specific health related quality of life measure for adults and adolescents with cystic fibrosis. Thorax. 2000;55:946–54.
18. Heslop K. Cognitive behavioural therapy in cystic fibrosis. J R Soc Med. 2006;99:27–9.
19. Robinson WM, Ravilly S, Berde C, Wohl ME. End of life care in cystic fibrosis. Pediatrics. 1997;100:205–9.
20. Mitchell I, Nakielna E, Tullis E, Adair C. Cystic fibrosis: end stage care in Canada. Chest. 2000;118:80–4.
21. Philip JA, Gold M, Sutherland S, et al. End of life care in adults with cystic fibrosis. J Palliat Med. 2008;11:198–203.
22. Young AC, Wilson JW, Kotsimbos TC, Naughton MT. Randomised placebo controlled trial of non-invasive ventilation for hypercapnia in cystic fibrosis. Thorax. 2011;63:72–7.
23. Sood N, Paradowski LJ, Yankaskas JR. Outcomes of intensive care unit care in adults with cystic fibrosis. Am J Respir Crit Care Med. 2001;163:335–8.
24. Dellon EP, Leigh MW, Yankaskas JR, Noah TL. Effects of lung transplantation on inpatient end of life care in cystic fibrosis. J Cyst Fibros. 2007;6:396–402.
25. Braithwaite M, Philip J, Tranberg H, et al. End of life care in CF: patients, families and staff experience and unmet needs. J Cyst Fibros. 2011;10:253–7.
26. Sands D, Repetto T, Dupont LJ, Korzeniewska-Eksterowicz A, Catastini P, Madge S. End of life care for patients with cystic fibrosis. J Cyst Fibros. 2011;10:S37–44.

Chapter 11
Respiratory Care in Neuromuscular Disease

Stephen C. Bourke and Catherine O'Neill

Abstract A structured approach to respiratory care improves outcomes, including symptom control, quality of life, and survival, in patients with neuromuscular diseases such as amyotrophic lateral sclerosis and Duchenne muscular dystrophy. Assessment of respiratory function should include bulbar function, respiratory muscle function, and cough effectiveness. Chest physiotherapy techniques and cough-assist devices help in the clearance of secretions. Supportive treatments such as non-invasive ventilation and gastrostomy feeding improve symptoms, survival, and quality of life. Early involvement of palliative care clinicians assists with advance care planning and provision of optimal end of life care in a setting of choice including hospital, home, or hospice. Symptoms such as breathlessness, choking, and pain can be controlled using treatments such as oxygen, sputum clearance techniques, opioids, benzodiazepines, and hyoscine.

Keywords Motor neurone disease • Muscular dystrophy • Amyotrophic lateral sclerosis • Non-invasive ventilation • Cough assist devices • Gastrostomy feeding

The term neuromuscular disorder (NMD) covers a wide range of conditions, with substantial variation in the pattern and severity of consequent muscle weakness and the rate of progression. Individual conditions are typically rare and are often classified by the nature of the primary defect. An alternative approach is to group

S.C. Bourke, M.B. BCh (hons), Ph.D., FRCP (✉)
Department of Respiratory Medicine, North Tyneside General Hospital,
Rake Lane, North Shields, Tyne and Wear NE29 8NH, UK
e-mail: stephen.bourke@NHCT.nhs.uk

C. O'Neill, M.B.B.S., MRCP
Department of Palliative Medicine,
Wansbeck General Hospital, Northumberland, UK

St Oswald's Hospice, Newcastle upon Tyne, UK

S.J. Bourke, E.T. Peel (eds.), *Integrated Palliative Care of Respiratory Disease*,
DOI 10.1007/978-1-4471-2230-2_11, © Springer-Verlag London 2013

conditions according to their natural clinical history, into reversible (e.g., myasthenia gravis, Guillain-Barré syndrome), stable/slowly progressive (e.g., post-polio syndrome, myotonic dystrophy, glycogen storage diseases, congenital myopathies, and mitochrondrial myopathy), and rapidly progressive disorders (e.g., amyotrophic lateral sclerosis (ALS), also known as motor neurone disease in the UK, and Duchenne muscular dystrophy (DMD)). In some conditions, different subtypes show substantial differences in severity and rate of progression (e.g., spinal muscular atrophy (SMA) and Nemaline myopathy); without ventilatory support, most children born with SMA type 1 die from respiratory failure within 2 years, whilst those with type 2 typically survive into adult life before ventilatory support is required. People with SMA types 3 and 4 are unlikely to need long-term ventilation. In this chapter, we focus on the symptoms and signs of respiratory muscle weakness in NMD, the importance of co-existent bulbar weakness, monitoring of respiratory function, ventilatory support in both the acute and long-term setting, alternative palliative therapies and advance care planning. The role of assisted cough techniques is also discussed in Chap. 4. Particular attention will be given to progressive disorders that affect people in late adolescence or adult life and that are consequently most often encountered in the adult palliative care setting, notably ALS and DMD.

In generalized NMD, the respiratory muscles are rarely spared, and respiratory function is a strong predictor of quality of life [1] and survival [2, 3]. Chest wall deformity, including kyphoscoliosis, may contribute to the impairment in ventilation. In some conditions, symptomatic respiratory muscle weakness is a late feature, after the patient has been wheelchair-bound for several years (such as DMD). In other conditions, the onset of respiratory symptoms may be variable (e.g., ALS). In patients with an established diagnosis, careful monitoring of respiratory symptoms and function facilitates appropriate education and discussion with the patient about the role of assisted cough techniques, ventilatory support, alternative palliative therapies, and advance care planning. However, if the diagnosis has not been previously recognized, the first presentation may be respiratory failure.

Structured Respiratory Care

A structured approach to respiratory care improves outcomes, including reducing the risk of respiratory tract infections and need for emergency initiation of ventilation, and increasing the use of elective non-invasive ventilation [4, 5] with consequent improvements in symptom control, quality of life and survival [5–7]. The multidisciplinary team caring for a patient with NMD should include a respiratory physician (and/or anesthetist), a respiratory technician or physiologist, a physiotherapist with expertise in ventilatory support and assisted cough techniques, a gastroenterologist, and/or interventional radiologist with expertise in gastrostomy tube placement and a palliative care physician. Respiratory assessment should include assessment of both symptoms and function. The frequency of assessment is largely determined by the rate of disease progression (typically 3 monthly for ALS and 6 monthly for DMD, but the frequency of review should be tailored to the individual patient). Patients with NMD should receive both pneumococcal and annual influenza vaccines, unless otherwise contra-indicated. Pooling of saliva should be dealt with by pharmacological or physical means. If control is poor, alternative options include Botulinum toxin and radiotherapy to the salivary glands. If placement of a gastrostomy tube is considered appropriate, it is important to consider the degree of impairment and rate of deterioration in respiratory muscle function.

Symptoms and Signs of Respiratory Muscle Weakness

Breathlessness should be assessed on exertion, during activities of daily living, when talking and on change in posture. Breathlessness usually only becomes apparent when respiratory muscle weakness is moderate or severe, particularly if mobility is limited and the patient does not suffer from co-existent lung disease. Consequently, the severity of respiratory muscle weakness is often under-estimated clinically [8]. In rapidly progressive disorders such as ALS, the duration between the onset of symptoms such as orthopnea and death may be only a few weeks [6, 9], emphasizing the importance of monitoring respiratory function, rather than relying on symptoms alone. The effect of posture on breathlessness is dependent on the pattern as well as the severity of respiratory muscle weakness; diaphragmatic weakness causes breathlessness lying flat and when immersed in water, whilst weakness of the intercostal muscles, such as seen in SMA and spinal injuries, causes breathlessness sitting upright. When respiratory muscle weakness is generalized, the patient may be most comfortable semi-recumbent. Patients with bulbar weakness may have difficulty distinguishing the sensation of choking on lying flat from true orthopnea; such patients also perform volitional respiratory function tests poorly, such that the degree of respiratory impairment is often over-estimated.

During sleep, the problems related to respiratory muscle weakness are compounded by loss of the wakefulness drive to breathe, the mechanical disadvantages of supine posture and rapid eye movement (REM)-related suppression of intercostal and accessory respiratory muscles. Consequent hypoventilation, with or without co-existent central and obstructive apneas and hypopneas, leads to frequent arousals with sleep disruption. Sleep-related symptoms, including frequent awakenings, unrefreshing sleep, daytime sleepiness, lethargy, fatigue, poor concentration, and nightmares are common, but non-specific; discomfort related to the inability to turn, episodes of choking related to bulbar impairment or anxiety and depression may also cause sleep disruption. Both patients and clinicians may fail to recognize when such symptoms are due to respiratory muscle weakness, once again highlighting the importance of monitoring respiratory function. As respiratory muscle weakness progresses, carbon dioxide retention ensues; in the early stages this may only occur during sleep, correcting shortly after waking, but subsequently becomes persistent and progressive. Symptoms include headaches, worse on wakening, loss of appetite, confusion, and drowsiness, ultimately leading to coma and death. Episodes of acute decompensation may be triggered by a variety of causes, discussed below. Sudden unexpected death and death during sleep are recognized and may reflect cardiac involvement, arrhythmias related to acute oxygen desaturation or simply mucus plugging that the patient was unable to clear.

An effective cough is dependent on good inspiratory, expiratory, and laryngeal (bulbar) muscle function. Consequently, involvement of these muscle groups may present with an ineffective cough and difficulty clearing secretions. Bulbar weakness not only causes problems with speech and swallowing, but also compromises the patient's ability to protect their airway and may present with recurrent episodes of choking, aspiration, and lower respiratory tract infections.

Clinical signs of respiratory muscle weakness are usually only apparent when the impairment is severe and include increased respiratory rate, shallow breathing, weak cough, weak sniff, use of accessory muscles, reduced chest expansion, reduced breath sounds, and abdominal paradox (inward movement of the abdomen on inspiration). Signs specific to diaphragmatic weakness include abdominal paradox, most apparent when supine, and active contraction of expiratory muscles when upright or semi-reclined [10]. Whilst expiration is normally passive, some patients actively contract their expiratory muscles as an adaptive mechanism, reducing their lung volume below functional residual capacity at the end of expiration. Subsequently, passive descent of the diaphragm assists inspiration. In SMA types 1 and 2, weakness of the intercostal muscles with preserved diaphragmatic function presents with bell-shaped deformity of the chest and chest paradox. Once respiratory failure ensues, signs include central cyanosis, dilated veins, coarse tremor, bounding pulse, papilledema, confusion, and reduced level of consciousness.

Assessing Respiratory Function

The assessment of respiratory function should include (a) bulbar function (speech and swallowing, including aspiration risk), (b) respiratory muscle function, and (c) cough effectiveness (determined by inspiratory, expiratory, and bulbar function). To formally assess bulbar function, various clinical tools are available, including simple clinical scales [11], the bulbar sub-component of the ALS Functional rating scale [12], and the Norris Bulbar Score [13].

When assessing respiratory muscle function, it is important to first consider bulbar function; in patients with severe bulbar impairment, volitional tests are unreliable, even when an adapted anesthetic facemask is used to overcome problems with air leak [14]. In such patients, greater reliance should be placed on measures of gas exchange, such as daytime oxygen saturation (S_pO_2) with measurement of arterial blood gases if <95 % and nocturnal oximetry and transcutaneous $PaCO_2$.

In patients without severe bulbar impairment, most clinicians rely on simple noninvasive indices such as S_pO_2, spirometry, maximum inspiratory (MIP) and expiratory (MEP) pressures, and sniff nasal inspiratory pressure (SNIP). Spirometry is widely available, easy to perform, and offers good reproducibility. Both inspiratory and expiratory muscle weakness reduce vital capacity (VC), which is a strong prognostic index [3, 8], and may be used to guide initiation of ventilatory support. VC should be measured sitting and supine if possible; a fall of >20 % indicates diaphragmatic weakness and, compared to erect VC, supine VC is a better index of diaphragmatic function [15]. Compared to VC, measures of respiratory pressures, such as SNIP and MIP, are more sensitive indices of respiratory muscle strength [16], better predictors of survival [17], and show less variation at initiation of ventilatory support for symptomatic respiratory failure. The best non-invasive and invasive predictors of daytime $PaCO_2$ are SNIP and sniff transdiaphragmatic pressure respectively, whilst non-volitional indices, using electric or magnetic fields to maximally stimulate nerves, are more uncomfortable for patients and offer little or no clinical advantage [14]. In ALS, regular monitoring of respiratory muscle function has been shown to reduce emergency initiation of non-invasive ventilation (NIV), use of tracheostomy ventilation, and, in patients with preserved bulbar function, improve survival from diagnosis [5].

In patients with sleep-related symptoms, nocturnal oximetry, ideally combined with transcutaneous $PaCO_2$, provides a simple screening tool for nocturnal hypoventilation, which may be used to direct (early) NIV [18]. More detailed limited sleep studies or full polysomnography offer the advantage of characterizing co-existent obstructive and central apneas and hypopneas.

Cough effectiveness can be assessed by measurement of peak cough flow, which can in turn be used to direct initiation of assisted cough techniques. Both peak cough flow and bulbar impairment (Norris Bulbar Score) predict problems with ineffective cough during respiratory tract infections [13].

Volume Recruitment and Assisted Cough Techniques

Volume recruitment techniques include glossopharyngeal (frog) breathing and breath-stacking aided by use of an ambu-bag and one-way valve or volume targeted ventilator to inflate the lungs to maximum insufflation capacity. If bulbar and facial muscle weakness limits the patient's ability to make a tight seal with a mouth-piece, an unvented anesthetic facemask can be used instead. Regular volume recruitment assists airway clearance and reverses or prevents atelectasis, improving gas exchange. Cough-assist techniques are recommended once peak cough flow falls below 160 l/min or, during respiratory tract infections or following procedures requiring sedation or general anesthesia, 270 l/min. The first step is insufflation, followed by an abdominal or thoraco-abdominal thrust timed with the cough (abdominal thrusts should be avoided after a meal). Alternatively, a mechanical insufflation-exsufflation (MI-E) device (CoughAssist™) may be used; in comparison to other techniques, MI-E achieves a greater increase in peak cough flow [19] and better outcomes during lower respiratory tract infections [20]. Whilst MI-E is usually administered via a facemask, it can be provided by a mouth-piece or endotracheal/tracheostomy tube. One treatment consists of five insufflation-exsufflation cycles (typical pressures: +40 & −40 cmH$_2$O), usually combined with a thrust timed with the exsufflation. Compared to deep suctioning, including via a tracheostomy tube, MI-E is more effective and avoids airway trauma. MI-E is less effective in patients with severe bulbar impairment [21], although a Guedel airway may be used to prevent upper airway collapse during exsufflation in this group.

Ventilatory Support

Survival

In stable or slowly progressive NMD, NIV offers a substantial improvement in survival compared to historical controls [22, 23]; randomized controlled trials comparing NIV to no ventilation have not been performed and would be regarded as unethical.

In rapidly progressive NMD, the role of NIV has been studied more extensively. In DMD complicated by daytime hypercapnia, compared to both historical controls (Fig. 11.1) [7] and those who declined treatment [24], NIV improves survival by 5–10 years. A randomized controlled trial (RCT) in DMD showed that, compared to standard treatment, early NIV (normal daytime PaCO$_2$ at initiation) was associated with higher mortality, largely related to respiratory tract infections [25]. The incidence of respiratory tract infections was similar in both arms, but patients on NIV were less likely to receive invasive ventilation and most deaths occurred in patients managed at home. False security may have contributed to sub-optimal management. In contrast, a more recent RCT in patients with NMD (including DMD) or chest wall restriction showed that early intervention (nocturnal hypoventilation; transcutaneous PaCO$_2$ > 6.5 kPa (48.8 mmHg)) improved gas exchange compared to controls [18]. Patients who declined early NIV were more likely to require initiation of NIV in an emergency and, in the control arm, the mean time to initiation of NIV for symptoms/daytime hypercapnia was only 8.3 months. Of note, in the later study by Ward and colleagues, favoring early intervention, nocturnal hypoventilation was confirmed by transcutaneous PaCO$_2$.

In ALS, NIV improves survival compared to patients who declined or were intolerant of treatment [26, 27] and randomized [6] controls. The RCT showed a survival advantage of 7 months for patients with good bulbar function (Fig. 11.2); of note, patients were enrolled regardless of their views on life prolonging therapy or social situation and those with more rapid progression were more likely to meet criteria for randomization within the timeframe of the study. In non-randomized studies, median survival from initiation of NIV of 14.2–18 months has been reported [11, 27, 28] and may be a better estimate of survival in well-motivated patients. In both the RCT of long-term NIV [6] and a prospective study of the use of NIV and cough assist during episodes of acute decompensation [29], a survival advantage was seen only in patients without severe bulbar impairment. However, there is evidence that patients with severe bulbar impairment who tolerate NIV survive longer than those who do not [26]. In a separate study, compared to historical controls, patients with

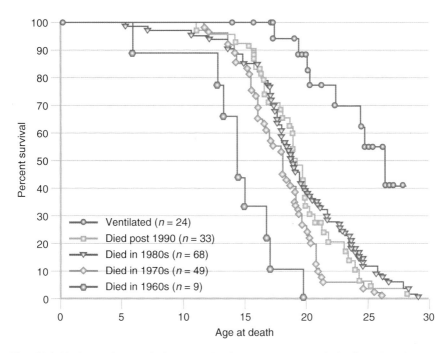

Fig. 11.1 Kaplan–Meier survival curves showing percentage survival of ventilated versus non-ventilated patients 1967–2002 [7]

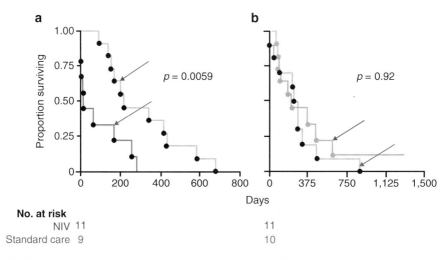

Fig. 11.2 Survival from randomization in a randomized controlled trial of non-invasive ventilation (*red*) compared to standard care (*blue*) in patients with amyotrophic lateral sclerosis and (**a**) normal or only moderately impaired bulbar function and (**b**) severe bulbar impairment [6]

severe bulbar impairment showed a survival advantage if they were hypercapnic, but not normocapnic, at the time of initiation [5]. This is biologically plausible; in such patients with poor airway protection, NIV may increase the risk of respiratory tract infections, but once daytime hypercapnia ensues, this risk may be outweighed by the benefits of ventilatory support. Compared to NIV, tracheostomy ventilation (TV) offers potentially longer survival, particularly if bulbar function is poor [30], but home care is less feasible.

The most important predictors of survival on NIV are adherence to treatment [11, 28] and bulbar function [11]. Good nutritional status [28], younger age, and good upper limb function [11] are also associated with a better outcome. In ALS, about 5 % of patients suffer from fronto-temporal dementia, which is associated with poor adherence to NIV and gastrostomy feeding, older age, and shorter survival.

Symptoms and Quality of Life (QoL)

Of 59 patients with NMD who were switched from TV to NIV, all expressed a preference for NIV, whilst 35 patients switched from NIV to TV expressed a significant preference for NIV for convenience, effect on speech, appearance, comfort and general acceptability, and equal preference for sleep, swallowing, and security [31].

In DMD, most patients on long-term ventilation are satisfied with their QoL. Whilst physical function is limited, aspects of QoL reflecting sleep-related symptoms, emotional and social function, and mental health scores are nearly normal and similar to patients not requiring ventilatory support [32].

In ALS, NIV improves sleep-related symptoms, social and emotional function, mental health, and general wellbeing. After correcting for side effects related to NIV, overall QoL and, in particular, sleep-related symptoms show a substantial improvement [6, 9]. Compared to patients with severe bulbar impairment, those with good bulbar function show larger improvements in symptom scores and QoL [6]. Most patients receiving NIV are cared for in their own home [33]. Compared to the carers of patients with similar physical limitation, but without respiratory impairment, carers of patients receiving NIV report similar QoL and strain [9]. Of interest, carers tend to significantly under-estimate the QoL experienced by the patient, whilst the patient tends to slightly over-estimate the QoL of their carer. Among patients receiving TV, the level of care and supervision required is much greater than that associated with NIV; consequently, home care is less feasible. The QoL of patients receiving TV in their own home is better than those in institutional care and similar to patients receiving NIV [33], but this is achieved at the expense of the QoL and burden experienced by their carers [30].

Patients may be afraid they may become trapped on a ventilator or, alternatively, will die a distressing death from suffocation. The latter concern was identified as one of the most important factors associated with the high rate of assisted suicide in patients with ALS in the Netherlands (ALS 20 %, cancer 5 %, and heart failure 0.5 %) [34]. It is important to reassure patients that if they elect to commence NIV, they will not become trapped on ventilation but rather this can be discontinued and effective alternative palliation provided if that is their wish. Symptoms such as breathlessness can be controlled and the reality is that most patients succumb peacefully to carbon dioxide narcosis. Palliation with opioids, sedatives, and oxygen therapy should not be commenced without first considering these issues and the role of ventilatory support.

Indications for NIV

In DMD, the results of two trials assessing early intervention (before daytime hypercapnia has ensued) showed conflicting results; the possible reasons for this are discussed above. In ALS, early initiation of NIV in patients with physiological impairment but no, or at most mild, symptoms is associated with higher overall NIV referral rates [35]. However, compared to standard criteria, adherence to NIV may be worse [11] and it is unclear whether early initiation confers an additional survival benefit; in patients with severe bulbar impairment the converse may be true [5]. A non-randomized trial reported that, compared to standard criteria for NIV, early intervention (VC≥65 % predicted) was associated with longer survival [36]. However, the interval between disease onset and initiation of NIV was similar in both arms, suggesting that the rate of progression was slower in the early intervention arm, which may, at least in part, explain the apparent survival advantage. The optimal timing of initiation of NIV in ALS in patients with and without severe bulbar impairment warrants further study. Currently recommended criteria for initiation of NIV in DMD and ALS [37] are shown in Boxes 11.1 and 11.2, respectively.

Box 11.1: Criteria for NIV in DMD
1. Signs or symptoms of hypoventilation (patients with (F)VC<30 % predicted are at especially high risk)[a]
2. Baseline SpO_2<95 % and/or blood or end-tidal $PaCO_2$>6 kPa (45 mmHg)[a]
3. An apnea-hypopnea index>10/h on polysomnography or four or more episodes of SpO_2<92 % or drops in SpO_2 of at least 4 %/h of sleep[a]
4. Nocturnal hypoventilation: $P_{TC}CO_2$>6.5 kPa (48.8 mmHg)[b]

[a]Bushby et al. [38]
[b]Ward et al. [18]

Box 11.2a: Criteria for NIV in ALS Without Severe Bulbar Impairment
1. (F)VC<50 % of predicted
2. (F)VC<80 % of predicted plus any symptoms or signs of respiratory impairment
3. SNIP or MIP<40 cmH_2O

4. SNIP or MIP <65 cmH$_2$O for men or 55 cmH$_2$O for women plus any symptoms or signs of respiratory impairment
5. Rate of decrease of SNIP or MIP of more than 10 cmH$_2$O per 3 months
6. Nocturnal hypoventilation

   (a) SpO$_2$ <90 % for >5 % of the night
   (b) P$_{TC}$CO$_2$ >6.5 kPa (48.8 mmHg)

7. Daytime hypercapnia (urgent referral)

Box 11.2b: Criteria for NIV in ALS with Severe Bulbar Impairment
1. Daytime hypercapnia (PaCO$_2$ >6 kPa (45 mmHg))
2. Nocturnal hypoventilation

   (a) SpO$_2$ <90 % for >5 % of the night
   (b) P$_{TC}$CO$_2$ >6.5 kPa (48.8 mmHg)

Abbreviations: (*F*)*VC* (forced) vital capacity, *SpO$_2$* oxygen saturation measured by pulse oximeter, *PaCO$_2$* partial pressure of carbon dioxide, *PTCCO$_2$* transcutaneous PaCO$_2$, *SNIP* sniff nasal inspiratory pressure, *MIP* maximum inspiratory pressure

Timing of Gastrostomy

Aspiration due to bulbar impairment, breathlessness during eating due to respiratory muscle weakness, and difficulty eating independently due to limb weakness may contribute to poor nutrition and weight loss. In the early stages, safe swallowing techniques, thickening of fluids and nutritional supplements may suffice. Placement of a gastrostomy tube improves survival [39] and should be considered if, despite these measures, the patient is failing to maintain adequate intake, has difficulty swallowing, and eating is tiring and/or has an unsafe swallow.

Percutaneous endoscopic gastrostomy (PEG) tube placement under conscious sedation is associated with a high complication rate in patients with VC <50 % [39, 40]. In patients with a rapid decline in respiratory function, early placement should be considered. In those with established severe respiratory muscle weakness (VC <50 %, P$_I$max/SNIP <40 % predicted/40 cmH$_2$O, daytime or nocturnal hypercapnia), radiologically guided insertion of a gastrostomy (RIG) tube may be a safer option; sedation is not required, the patient does not have to lie completely flat, and it is easier to provide support with NIV [41]. Alternatively, PEG insertion may be performed either with NIV support (with increased pressure support and FiO$_2$ to overcome airleak) or intubation and ventilation, followed by extubation onto NIV. Of importance, complications include diaphragmatic splinting and pneumonia, and most deaths occur after, not during, the procedure [40, 41]; post-procedure respiratory care is important, including volume recruitment, cough assist, and, if required, NIV.

Acute Decompensation

Patients with NMD may present in extremis with acute, or acute on chronic, respiratory failure. Such episodes may be triggered by posture, injudicious use of uncontrolled oxygen therapy [42] or sedatives, mucus plugging, episodes of aspiration, respiratory tract infections, or pneumonia [29]. Of note, even upper respiratory tract infections are associated with a decline in respiratory muscle function. Whilst decompensation may be triggered by a reversible precipitant, most patients also have severe respiratory muscle weakness and, if they survive, will require long-term ventilatory support, particularly if the underlying condition is ALS or DMD [29] rather than a more slowly progressive disorder [43]. Consequently, when deciding whether or not acute ventilatory support is appropriate, and if so, how this should be provided, all factors influencing the outcome of both acute and long-term support, and the acceptability of this to the patient, should be borne in mind. The decision to commence ventilatory support may have to be made in an emergency, often by clinicians with limited knowledge of the underlying NMD; where possible it is preferable to discuss such issues with patients in advance and clarify their views. Structured respiratory care, including regular monitoring of respiratory function, reduces the need for emergency initiation of ventilation [5] but this is not entirely avoidable; unfortunately some patients present in acute respiratory failure before a diagnosis has been made.

In patients without severe bulbar impairment, compared to invasive ventilation, non-invasive ventilation reduces length of stay in intensive care and complications such as ventilator-associated pneumonia and may improve survival [29, 44]. Compared to intubation, communication is better preserved using non-invasive support, facilitating subsequent discussions with the patient about their care, including long-term support. In addition to providing ventilatory support, it is also important to assist clearance of secretions [29, 44]. Use of MI-E devices achieves better secretion clearance than deep suctioning and is preferable to mini-tracheostomy. Complications such as surgical emphysema are avoided and insufflation helps volume recruitment. Mucolytics, such as nebulized N-acetylcysteine 1–2 g, can be helpful. If a patient has been intubated to assist transfer between units, they can be extubated onto NIV. Those who have been inappropriately tracheostomized can also be converted to NIV once they are clinically stable [31]. If bulbar function is severely impaired, the patient is unlikely to survive the acute episode using non-invasive ventilation and cough assist alone [29]. If long-term TV is acceptable to the patient, they should be offered invasive ventilation; otherwise alternative palliation may be more appropriate.

Current Use of NIV

There has been a progressive increase in the proportion of patients with NMD treated with NIV over the last 10–15 years [4, 7, 35] A recent UK survey of respiratory care in ALS [35] showed that, compared to 2000, the proportions of patients referred for, and successfully established on, NIV have increased 2.6 and 3.4 fold, respectively. The most common deterrents to NIV referral were cognitive impairment, social isolation, rapid disease progression, and severe bulbar impairment. The neurologists who referred the most patients were more likely to monitor respiratory function regularly, measure respiratory pressures and arterial blood gases, consider early intervention, and rely on a combination of symptoms and physiological impairment to guide referral, reflecting the UK National Institute of Clinical Excellence (NICE) guidelines [37]. Wider application of NICE guidelines is likely to reduce variation in respiratory care and further improve the assessment of patients and use of NIV.

Recognizing the Terminal Phase in Progressive Neuromuscular Disease

In most neuromuscular conditions, currently available therapies have either no or only limited effect on the underlying disease process. Supportive treatments such as NIV and gastrostomy feeding improve survival in appropriately selected patients, but do not prevent progressive disability. The primary aim of most treatments is palliative; to optimize symptom control and improve quality of life.

In patients with progressive NMD, respiratory failure is the most common cause of death. However, as discussed above, symptoms are often only recognized at a late stage. Consequently, the degree of impairment in, and rate of decline of, respiratory function is key to anticipating the end stage of the condition [45]. Both within and between different NMDs, there is substantial variation in the rate of decline in respiratory muscle function, although within an individual patient the trajectory tends to be more consistent. Whilst there is often a gradual deterioration and a worsening of symptoms over the final few weeks and months of life, some patients deteriorate very quickly and die suddenly or within a few days [46]. Identifying when someone with a neuromuscular condition may be approaching the end of life can be very challenging. However, there are several indicators that may suggest the disease is progressing and trigger end of life discussions and planning (see Box 11.3).

Box 11.3: Indicators of Disease Progression in Neuromuscular Conditions
Decline in respiratory function
Swallowing problems

Recurring lower respiratory tract infections
First episode of aspiration pneumonia
Marked decline in physical status
Cognitive impairment
Weight loss
Significant complex symptoms
Recurring hospital admissions

Adapted from End of life care in long term neurological conditions: a framework for implementation

Regular assessment, tailored to the individual patient, is essential to ensure early recognition of the onset of the terminal phase of the condition. Clearly, there may be occasions when there is a reversible component to an observed deterioration in a person's condition, which may respond to appropriate treatment if recognized. This may include inter-current infections, an underlying psychological condition such as depression, or an adverse response to medication changes or increases. Furthermore, despite disease progression, survival may be extended by non-invasive and tracheostomy ventilation and gastrostomy feeding. However, not all patients desire treatment measures that may extend their life in the face of progressive disability. Therefore, sensitive and appropriately timed discussions with patients and their families are essential to try and clarify patient wishes in advance.

Advance Care Planning in Neuromuscular Diseases

Optimal timing for end of life discussions in neuromuscular conditions such as ALS is described in the international literature [47]. Several triggers for the potential introduction of such discussions with patients and their families have been suggested (see Box 11.4).

Box 11.4: Triggers for Initiating End of Life Discussions
1. The patient opens the discussion for end of life information and/or interventions
2. Severe psychological and/or social or spiritual distress or suffering
3. Pain requiring high dosages of analgesic medications
4. Dysphagia requiring feeding tube
5. Meeting criteria for ventilatory support (see Box 11.2 above)
6. Loss of function in two body regions (regions include bulbar, arms, and legs)

Adapted from Bede et al. [47]

With the recent evolution of advance care planning and the increasingly earlier involvement of palliative care teams in the care of patients with NMDs, such discussions may occur earlier and more frequently. Discussions may lead to the development of an advance statement, an advance decision to refuse treatment (ADRT), or the appointment of a person with Lasting Power of Attorney for health and welfare (see Chap. 13).

In patients with neuromuscular conditions, advance care planning may play an important role in directing symptom management, especially in the last days and hours of life, and prevent life-prolonging treatments being instigated or continued contrary to their actual preferences. Of importance, at the time an advance care plan is prepared, the patient must be competent, able to process relevant information, and display an appropriate appreciation of the potential consequences of any decisions made [47].

Discontinuation of Non-invasive Ventilation in Neuromuscular Disease

Early discussions with patients and relatives around end of life issues in the terminal phase of NMDs, such as the discontinuation of non-invasive ventilation and the use of documented advance statements are essential for patient-centered decision making [48]. The ability to maintain control over decisions regarding ventilation and in particular its discontinuation is fundamental to patients deliberating over whether to commence ventilation [49].

As neuromuscular disease progresses, patients established on NIV may find that they become increasingly dependent on the ventilator to relieve symptoms of breathlessness, sometimes requiring it up to 24 h/day. During the terminal phase, ventilated patients may find ongoing treatment brings little hope of recovery, but instead prolongs the dying process. It may be appropriate to consider or offer alternative measures to relieve breathlessness (both non-pharmacological and pharmacological) in order to allow patients periods of freedom from the ventilator.

However, the patient may ask for ventilation to be discontinued altogether, with adequate symptom control to minimize any associated distress [46]. In the event that a competent patient who is deemed to have mental capacity and is not suffering from a depressive disorder or a patient with a valid and applicable ADRT requests discontinuation of non-invasive ventilation, then such wishes should and must be respected. Continuation of ventilation, against a patient's will, would be both ethically and legally indefensible. Elective withdrawal of ventilator support can cause distress and anxiety to all involved and requires sensitive and thoughtful discussion, with patient, relatives, and healthcare professionals [46].

In the event that non-invasive ventilation is to be withdrawn, a multidisciplinary team approach is important. The patient, primary carer, and family should be central to all discussions and preparation. Palliative care services are often already involved. This is important in terms of facilitating relationships and rapport prior to the terminal phase during which palliative care input is very valuable.

A staged withdrawal of ventilation, also referred to as *terminal weaning*, is usually advocated. Timed back-up breaths should be disabled and the level of ventilatory support is typically reduced over several minutes or hours. The ventilator settings should be adjusted to maintain symptomatic relief, whilst simultaneously allowing gradual hypercapnia to develop [50]. Premedication with sedatives and opioids should be administered prior to commencement of weaning from the ventilator, particularly in conscious individuals. Midazolam at a dose of 2.5–5 mg subcutaneously, as a stat dose (may require higher doses if already receiving regular sedation) should be administered, together with an anti-secretory agent and/or opioid medication if secretions, discomfort, or breathlessness are present. The effect of these medications should be assessed within 30 min and repeated if necessary, prior to reduction of the ventilator settings. Further medications should be administered and titrated as appropriate, according to patients' symptoms and responses. This staged ventilatory withdrawal allows for rapid identification and treatment of any distress or worsening symptoms that may occur after each adjustment of the ventilator [50]. It may be appropriate to commence a continuous subcutaneous infusion of opioids, benzodiazepines, and anti-secretory medications if frequent stat doses are required. This management strategy should not pose any ethical dilemmas; the primary aim of care is to relieve symptoms and distress, rather than to prolong life. If managed appropriately, most patients become progressively more drowsy, then unconscious, due to increasing hypercapnia and die peacefully [51].

Role of Palliative Care in Patients with Neuromuscular Disease

The aim of palliative care is to relieve symptoms and to provide psychosocial and spiritual support, thereby optimizing the quality of life of both patients and their families, whilst minimizing obstacles to a peaceful death and supporting the family through the bereavement process [50]. The recent expansion of palliative care into non-malignant disease has helped improve symptom control and quality of life for patients and support for carers in progressive neuromuscular conditions such as ALS [52]. Given the progressive nature of neuromuscular conditions and the limited treatments available, it is largely accepted that management from diagnosis is palliative with the aim of optimizing symptoms and quality of life [45]. It has been widely recommended that optimal management should incorporate a multidisciplinary approach, with evidence supporting an improvement in both quality of life and survival in patients with ALS managed in a multidisciplinary care setting [53]. This should include early involvement of palliative care which can help to facilitate and support preparation and anticipation of disease progression and the provision of optimal end of life care. This consequently allows better standards of care and an improved quality of life for both the patients and their families [45, 46]. The development of respiratory muscle weakness in patients with NMD is a poor prognostic sign. It is strongly encouraged that patients are offered referral to specialist palliative care services at this stage, if this has not already occurred [48]. Such a multidisciplinary approach to the care of patients with NMDs facilitates both symptom control measures and psychosocial support, as well as consideration of more "active" management options, such as assisted ventilation, dependent on individual patient preferences [46].

Common End of Life Symptoms in Advanced Neuromuscular Diseases and Their Management

General Principles: Symptom Control

A multidisciplinary approach to the management of patients with end-stage neuromuscular diseases is essential. All patients should have access to specialist palliative care in a setting of their choice, including hospital, community, or hospice. An essential aspect of optimal end of life care for patients with advanced NMD should include anticipatory preparation, both in terms of communication and the provision and availability of medications, in the event of a rapid decline. Key drugs should be made available, in all care settings.

The Just in Case (JIC) Kit was introduced in the United Kingdom by the Motor Neurone Disease Association in 1991 (previously called the Breathing Space Kit) [54]. The JIC Kit is part of a programme that facilitates discussion about end of life care in ALS for patients, families, and healthcare professionals. It provides written information and includes a box containing a range of medications. These can be used in the event of a sudden deterioration in the person with ALS who is intolerant of, has declined, or who wishes to withdraw from NIV. In particular, it is aimed at alleviating symptoms such as choking, breathlessness, and associated panic, which commonly occur at the end of life. The JIC Kit is supplied on a named patient basis to the general practitioner free of charge. The main classes of drugs included are opioid, sedative, and anticholinergic agents. This programme helps to facilitate advance care planning by initiating discussions around the possibility of deterioration and how this would be managed were it to occur [55].

Patients with advanced neuromuscular diseases may experience a range of both physical and psychological symptoms as well as social and spiritual problems. Common symptoms at the end of life include dyspnea, pain, and distress. Both patients and their carers are often concerned that the end of life may be a very distressing process. Some patients express fears about dying from choking or with uncontrolled pain. However, although choking sensations may occur in NMD, both death from choking and death with severe, uncontrolled pain are extremely rare. Evidence shows that with access to palliative care, distress at the end of life is rare and that the provision of good symptom control measures facilitates a peaceful death in the majority of patients [51].

Physical Symptoms at the End of Life

Breathlessness

The majority of patients with progressive NMDs die from respiratory failure due to respiratory muscle weakness. Symptoms of ventilatory failure, including progressive breathlessness, develop insidiously in the later stages of the disease. Breathlessness is common, affecting up to 85 % patients in the terminal phase [55].

Oxygen Therapy

Prior to the terminal phase, uncontrolled oxygen should be avoided as it can lead to potentially fatal carbon dioxide retention, with associated symptoms, such as headache and increased drowsiness. At the end of life, the risks associated with oxygen therapy may be outweighed by the need for effective symptom control. Hypoxia causes greater distress than hypercapnia and oxygen may be used to provide symptomatic relief. However, where appropriate, the patient should be made aware of this potential risk. In the cancer setting, oxygen is generally better than air in severely hypoxic patients ($SaO_2 < 90$ %) [56]. However, with lesser degrees of hypoxia or with normal oxygen saturation levels, there is no difference in the benefit achieved with oxygen or piped air delivered by nasal prongs [57]. This suggests that it may be the sensation of airflow plus the cooling effect, rather than the oxygen itself, that provides symptomatic relief in many patients [58]. It may therefore be useful to encourage patients to try the benefit of an open window or fan, before trying oxygen.

Opioids

Strong opioids, such as morphine sulphate, reduce the ventilatory response to hypercapnia and hypoxia, thereby reducing respiratory effort and breathlessness. High-dose opioids in a opioid-naive patient, or a rapid escalation in dose, may potentially cause respiratory decompensation, particularly if combined with benzodiazepines or uncontrolled oxygen. In the cancer and COPD setting, evidence supports an improvement in breathlessness at doses that do not cause respiratory depression [59, 60]. In these settings, and when used competently and appropriately, with gradual and individual dose titration, there is no evidence that strong opioids shorten life. Whilst there is evidence to support the safe use of strong opioids for chronic pain in patients with ALS [61], concerns still remain regarding the potential risks of using strong opioids for the acute relief of breathlessness at the end of life in these patients. As with the use of uncontrolled oxygen, the risk versus benefit balance has to be carefully assessed. The priority at this stage in the disease trajectory remains the optimization of symptoms and minimization of suffering which may be achieved through the cautious and gradual titration of strong opioids.

In patients with NMD, strong opioids are often used to control symptoms of pain and breathlessness, well in advance of the terminal phase of the illness. In patients who are already using morphine for pain, a dose of 25–100 % of the 4-hourly (instant release) analgesic dose may be needed, depending on the degree of breathlessness. However, in opioid-naive patients, small doses of immediate release morphine should be used initially, such as 2.5 mg orally, as required. If more than two doses are required within a 24 h period, morphine should be prescribed regularly (either short- or long-acting morphine) and titrated according to response, duration of effect, and adverse effects. If the oral or per gastrostomy route is not possible, patients may benefit from having a continuous subcutaneous infusion of morphine, which is sometimes better tolerated and may provide greater relief by avoiding the peaks and troughs of oral medication. The same principles should be applied to the use of alternative strong opioids.

Benzodiazepines

In NMDs, benzodiazepines are commonly used, often in conjunction with strong opioids, in the management of symptomatic breathlessness. In contrast to opioids, benzodiazepines probably do not have a specific anti-breathlessness effect [57]. A recent Cochrane review concluded that currently there is no evidence that benzodiazepines relieve breathlessness in patients with advanced cancer and COPD [62]. Benzodiazepines caused more drowsiness as an adverse effect compared to placebo, but less compared to morphine. The authors recommend considering benzodiazepines as a second- or third-line treatment within an individual therapeutic trial, when opioids and non-pharmacological measures have failed to control breathlessness. Nevertheless, there is a proven association between breathlessness and anxiety and therefore reducing anxiety may help to lessen the sensation of breathlessness and help patients to cope with it more effectively. As discussed above, benzodiazepines are also useful during withdrawal of ventilation.

Patients with severe respiratory compromise at the end of life may experience distressing breathlessness associated with high levels of anxiety. In these patients, the use of medications such as benzodiazepines to alleviate distressing breathlessness and its associated anxiety may result in impaired respiratory effort. In those patients who retain capacity, it may be appropriate to advise them of the potential risks associated with such treatment. For those patients who lack capacity, a decision to use such medications should be made by the multidisciplinary team caring for the patient, in the best interests of the patient and involving family members and carers sensitively, in the decision-making process. At this stage in the disease trajectory and in the presence of such distressing symptoms, the aim of treatment must be to optimize comfort and to minimize distress, even if this *potentially* risks shortening an already very short prognosis [50].

Secretions

Retention of upper airway secretions in patients with bulbar impairment commonly occurs in advance of the terminal phase in conditions such as ALS. However, as any severely unwell patient approaches the end of life, they become less conscious and less able to cough and clear respiratory secretions, which can accumulate in the upper airways and result in noisy breathing. Whilst this may be very distressing for family members and healthcare professionals to witness, the patient is generally not aware or distressed because of the diminished level of consciousness. Hence, treatment of this symptom is usually for the benefit of those caring for the patient. It is good practice to anticipate and treat early as once upper airway secretions become established, they are more difficult to manage. Measures include both non-pharmacological, including reassurance to family members, positional changes to aid postural drainage, assisted cough techniques (including MI-E), and oropharyngeal or tracheal suction. Drugs such as hyoscine hydrobromide, hyoscine butylbromide, and glycopyrronium have similar efficacy in reducing secretions as detailed in Appendix B [57].

Pain

Pain occurs commonly throughout the disease trajectory of many neuromuscular conditions, affecting up to 73 % patients during the disease progression in ALS [55]. Pain from neuromuscular disease is usually multifactorial in nature and includes musculoskeletal, skin pressure and muscle spasm, and spasticity-related pain. Consequently, pain management has often been instigated well in advance of the terminal phase of the condition. Nevertheless, pain is a common symptom at the end of life, occurring in 70–76 % patients dying from ALS at home and in the hospice setting [55].

The majority of pain management in NMDs, such as ALS, has been adopted from experience in other fields, including cancer and general pain literature. The principles of pain management in NMD are based on the WHO analgesic ladder [63] which facilitates gradual, step by step progression from simple analgesia to weak, followed by strong opioids, together with adjuncts. Many patients with NMD may require regular administration of strong opioid analgesics to control their pain adequately. This can be administered in a variety of ways, including the oral, gastrostomy, transdermal, or subcutaneous routes.

In the advanced phase of the disease and in the presence of a gastrostomy, the administration of analgesia can continue as normal, although dose escalation may be required. In the absence of a gastrostomy, patients may require an alternative route of administration to ensure optimal ongoing pain control and the avoidance of opioid withdrawal. The subcutaneous route is used extensively in palliative care, in patients for whom the oral route has become increasingly difficult or impossible. In patients already established on regular oral strong opioids, this can be converted to (the equivalent dose of) a continuous subcutaneous infusion, delivered by a portable syringe driver. Breakthrough pain relief can be administered by stat doses of analgesia via subcutaneous injections, the dose of which is determined by the background analgesic dose (i.e., 1/10–1/6 of the 24-h background analgesic dose).

Psychological Symptoms

Anxiety/Agitation

Anxiety can become marked when respiratory insufficiency occurs. It can manifest in several ways, both physical and psychological. During the terminal phase of neuromuscular conditions, such as ALS, a generalized restlessness is not uncommon. Management will depend upon the underlying cause, as well as the stage in the disease trajectory. It is good practice to try and identify and treat any potentially reversible causes, such as uncontrolled pain, constipation, or urinary retention. Benzodiazepines are commonly used during the terminal phase, for their anxiolytic and muscle-relaxant properties and their indirect effect on symptoms of breathlessness. They also have a sedating effect, which is desired by some patients during this phase. Lorazepam (oral or sublingual) as required or regularly can be used in those patients who are able to take medications via the oral route. For those patients who are unable to swallow, subcutaneous midazolam (starting at 2.5 mg) is the drug of choice. This can be started on an as-required basis initially to assess effectiveness. If this provides good symptomatic relief, it may be appropriate to commence a continuous subcutaneous infusion via a syringe driver, titrated gradually according to symptoms.

References

1. Bourke S, Shaw P, Gibson G. Respiratory function vs sleep-disordered breathing as predictors of QOL in ALS. Neurology. 2001;57:2040–4.
2. Gay P, Westbrook P, Daube J, et al. Effects of alterations in pulmonary function and sleep variables on survival in patients with amyotrophic lateral sclerosis. Mayo Clin Proc. 1991;66:686–94.
3. Phillips M, Smith P, Carroll N, et al. Nocturnal oxygenation and prognosis in Duchenne muscular dystrophy. Am J Respir Crit Care Med. 1999;160:198–202.
4. Chio A, Calvo A, Moglia C, et al. Non-invasive ventilation in amyotrophic lateral sclerosis: a 10 year population based study. J Neurol Neurosurg Psychiatry. 2012;83:377–81.
5. Farrero E, Prats E, Povedano M, et al. Survival in amyotrophic lateral sclerosis with home mechanical ventilation. Chest. 2005;127:2132–8.
6. Bourke S, Tomlinson M, Williams T, et al. Effects of non-invasive ventilation on survival and quality of life in patients with amyotrophic lateral sclerosis: a randomised controlled trial. Lancet Neurol. 2006;5:140–7.

7. Eagle M, Baudouin S, Chandler C, et al. Survival in Duchenne muscular dystrophy: improvements in life expectancy since 1967 and the impact of home nocturnal ventilation. Neuromusc Disord. 2002;12:926–9.

8. Fallat R, Jewitt B, Bass M, et al. Spirometry in amyotrophic lateral sclerosis. Arch Neurol. 1979;36:74–80.

9. Mustfa N, Walsh E, Bryant V, et al. The effect of noninvasive ventilation on ALS patients and their caregivers. Neurology. 2006;66:1211–7.

10. Gibson G. Diaphragmatic paresis: pathophysiology, clinical features and investigation. Thorax. 1989;44:960–70.

11. Bourke S, Bullock R, Williams T, et al. Noninvasive ventilation in ALS: indications and effect on quality of life. Neurology. 2003;61:171–7.

12. Cedarbaum J, Stambler N, Malta E, et al. The ALSFRS-R: a revised ALS functional rating scale that incorporates assessments of respiratory function. BDNF ALS Study Group (Phase III). J Neurol Sci. 1999;169:13–21.

13. Sancho J, Servera E, Díaz J, et al. Predictors of ineffective cough during a chest infection in patients with stable amyotrophic lateral sclerosis. Am J Respir Crit Care Med. 2007;175:1266–71.

14. Lyall R, Donaldson N, Polkey M, et al. Respiratory muscle strength and ventilatory failure in amyotrophic lateral sclerosis. Brain. 2000;124:2000–13.

15. Lechtzin N, Wiener C, Shade D, et al. Spirometry in the supine position improves the detection of diaphragmatic weakness in patients with amyotrophic lateral sclerosis. Chest. 2002;121:436–42.

16. De Troyer A, Borenstein S, Cordier R. Analysis of lung volume restriction in patients with respiratory muscle weakness. Thorax. 1980;35:603–10.

17. Morgan R, McNally S, Alexander M, et al. Use of sniff nasal-inspiratory force to predict survival in amyotrophic lateral sclerosis. Am J Respir Crit Care Med. 2005;171:269–74.

18. Ward S, Chatwin M, Heather S, et al. Randomised controlled trial of non-invasive ventilation (NIV) for nocturnal hypoventilation in neuromuscular and chest wall disease patients with daytime normocapnia. Thorax. 2005;60:1019–24.

19. Chatwin M, Ross E, Hart N, et al. Cough augmentation with mechanical insufflation/exsufflation in patients with neuromuscular weakness. Eur Respir J. 2003;21:502–8.

20. Vianello A, Corrado A, Arcaro G, et al. Mechanical insufflation-exsufflation improves outcomes for neuromuscular disease patients with respiratory tract infections. Am J Phys Med Rehabil. 2005;84:83–8.

21. Sancho J, Servera E, Diaz J, et al. Efficacy of mechanical insufflation-exsufflation in medically stable patients with amyotrophic lateral sclerosis. Chest. 2004;125:1400–5.

22. Simonds A, Elliott M. Outcome of domiciliary nasal intermittent positive pressure ventilation in restrictive and obstructive disorders. Thorax. 1995;50:604–9.

23. Nugent A, Smith I, Shneerson J. Domicilliary-assisted ventilation in patients with myotonic dystrophy. Chest. 2002;121:459–65.

24. Vianello A, Bevilacqua M, Salvador V, et al. Long-term nasal intermittent positive pressure ventilation in advanced Duchenne's muscular dystrophy. Chest. 1994;105:445–8.

25. Raphael J, Chevret S, Chastang C, et al. Randomised trial of preventive nasal ventilation in Duchenne muscular dystrophy. French Multicentre Cooperative Group on Home Mechanical Ventilation Assistance in Duchenne de Boulogne Muscular Dystrophy. Lancet. 1994;343:1600–4.

26. Aboussouan L, Khan S, Meeker D, et al. Effect of noninvasive positive-pressure ventilation on survival in amyotrophic lateral sclerosis. Ann Intern Med. 1997;127:450–3.

27. Kleopa K, Sherman M, Neal B, et al. Bipap improves survival and rate of pulmonary function decline in patients with ALS. J Neurol Sci. 1999;164:82–8.

28. Lo Coco D, Marchese S, Pesco M, et al. Noninvasive positive-pressure ventilation in ALS: predictors of tolerance and survival. Neurology. 2006;67:761–5.

29. Servera E, Sancho J, Zafra M, et al. Alternatives to endotracheal intubation for patients with neuromuscular diseases. Am J Phys Med Rehabil. 2005;84:851–7.

30. Marchese S, Lo Coco D, Lo Coco A. Outcome and attitudes toward home tracheostomy ventilation of consecutive patients: a 10-year experience. Respir Med. 2008;102:430–6.

31. Bach J. A comparison of long-term ventilatory support alternatives from the perspective of the patient and care giver. Chest. 1993;104:1702–6.
32. Kohler M, Clarenbach C, Boni L, et al. Quality of life, physical disability, and respiratory impairment in Duchenne muscular dystrophy. Am J Respir Crit Care Med. 2005;172:1032–6.
33. Moss A, Oppenheimer E, Casey P, et al. Patients with amyotrophic lateral sclerosis receiving long-term mechanical ventilation: advance care planning and outcomes. Chest. 1996;110:249–55.
34. Maessen M, Veldink J, Van den Berg L, et al. Requests for euthanasia: origin of suffering in ALS, heart failure, and cancer patients. J Neurol. 2010;257:1192–8.
35. O'Neill C, Williams T, Peel E, et al. Non-invasive ventilation in motor neuron disease: an update of current UK practice. J Neurol Neurosurg Psychiatry. 2012;83:371–6.
36. Lechtzin N, Scott Y, Busse A, et al. Early use of non-invasive ventilation prolongs survival in subjects with ALS. Amyotroph Lateral Scler. 2007;8:185–8.
37. NICE. Motor neurone disease – non-invasive ventilation. London: National Institute for Health and Clinical Excellence; 2010.
38. Bushby K, et al. Diagnosis and management of Duchenne muscular dystrophy, part 2: implementation of multidisciplinary care. Lancet Neurol. 2010;9:177–89.
39. Mazzini L, Corra T, Zaccala M, et al. Percutaneous endoscopic gastrostomy and enteral nutrition in amyotrophic lateral sclerosis. J Neurol. 1995;242:695–8.
40. Kasarskis E, Scarkata D, Hill R, et al. A retrospective study of percutaneous endoscopic gastrostomy in ALS patients during the BDNF and CNTF trials. J Neurol Sci. 1999;169: 118–25.
41. Lewis D, Ampong M, Rio A, et al. Mushroom-cage gastrostomy tube placement in patients with amyotrophic lateral sclerosis: a 5-year experience in 104 patients in a single institution. Eur Radiol. 2009;19:1763–71.
42. Gay P, Edmonds L. Severe hypercapnia after low-flow oxygen therapy in patients with neuromuscular disease and diaphragmatic dysfunction. Mayo Clin Proc. 1995;70:327–30.
43. Banerjee S, Licence V, Oscroft N, et al. Outcome after prolonged invasive mechanical ventilation in myotonic dystrophy. Thorax. 2011;66:A179.
44. Vianello A, Bevilacqua M, Arcaro G, et al. Non-invasive ventilatory approach to treatment of acute respiratory failure in neuromuscular disorders. A comparison with endotracheal intubation. Intensive Care Med. 2000;26:384–90.
45. Oliver D, Borasio G, Walsh D. Palliative care in amytrophic lateral sclerosis – from diagnosis to bereavement. 2nd ed. Oxford: Oxford University Press; 2006.
46. Oliver D, Campbell C, Wright A. Palliative care of patients with motor neurone disease. Prog Palliat Care. 2007;15:285–93.
47. Bede P, Oliver D, Stodart J, et al. Palliative care in amyotrophic lateral sclerosis: a review of current international guidelines and initiatives. J Neurol Neurosurg Psychiatry. 2011;82: 413–8.
48. Eng D. Management guidelines for motor neurone disease patients on non-invasive ventilation at home. Palliat Med. 2006;20:69–79.
49. Young J, Marshall C, Anderson E. Amyotrophic lateral sclerosis patients' perspectives on use of mechanical ventilation. Health Soc Work. 1994;19:253–60.
50. Oliver D, Borasio G, Walsh D. Palliative care in amytrophic lateral sclerosis. Oxford: Oxford University Press; 2000.
51. Neudert C, Oliver D, Wasner M, et al. The course of the terminal phase in patients with amyotrophic lateral sclerosis. J Neurol. 2001;248:612–6.
52. Veronese S, Gallo G, Valle A. Specialist Palliative Care service for people severely affected by neurodegenerative conditions: does this make a difference to palliative care outcomes? Results of Nepal – an explorative randomised control trial. Palliat Med. 2010;24:S25–6.
53. Van den Berg J, Kalmijn S, Lindeman E, et al. Multidisciplinary ALS care improves quality of life in patients with ALS. Neurology. 2005;65:1264–7.
54. MNDA. Just in case kit. 2012. Available from http://www.mndassociation.org/for_professionals/association_resources/jic_kit.html.

55. Oliver D. The quality of care and symptom control – the effects on the terminal phase of ALS/MND. J Neurol Sci. 1996;139(Suppl):134–6.
56. Bruera E, Sweeney C, Willey J, et al. A randomized controlled trial of supplemental oxygen versus air in cancer patients with dyspnea. Palliat Med. 2003;17:659–63.
57. Twycross R, Wilcock A, StarkToller C. Symptom management in advanced cancer. 4th ed. Nottingham: Palliativedrugs.com Ltd; 2002.
58. Kerr D. A bedside fan for terminal dyspnoea. Am J Hosp Care. 1989;6:22.
59. Bruera E, Macmillan K, Pither J, et al. Effects of morphine on the dyspnea of terminal cancer patients. J Pain Symptom Manage. 1990;5:341–4.
60. Jennings A, Davies A, Higgins J, et al. A systematic review of the use of opioids in the management of dyspnoea. Thorax. 2002;57:939–44.
61. Oliver D. Opioid medication in the palliative care of motor neurone disease. Palliat Med. 1998;12:113–5.
62. Simon S, Higginson I, Booth S, et al. Benzodiazepines for the relief of breathlessness in advanced malignant and non-malignant diseases in adults. Cochrane Database of Systematic Reviews 2010, Issue 1. Art. No.: CD007354. DOI:10.1002/14651858.CD007354.pub2.
63. World Health Organisation. Cancer pain relief and palliative care: report of a WHO Expert Committee. Geneva; 1990.

Chapter 12
Palliative Care in the Intensive Care Unit

Alistair D. Gascoigne and Stephen J. Bourke

Abstract The intensive care unit (ICU) is a setting in which critically ill patients receive high-intensity treatments such as mechanical ventilation to sustain life. These patients are at high risk of dying such that ICU clinicians manage dying patients and their families on a daily basis. ICU care is associated with a high level of symptoms and palliation of suffering is important throughout the course of treatment. Treatment is inherently intrusive and some patients with advanced disease may not wish to undergo ICU care, particularly if their deterioration indicates progression of their disease rather than a reversible complication. Failed ICU care may impose additional suffering and detract from the end of life experience. It is important to recognize when treatment is merely prolonging the dying phase. The focus then switches to making the dying process comfortable and dignified. Intrusive treatments are withdrawn and opioids and benzodiazepines are used to relieve distress. Because of the severity of the illness, the dying phase is often short, over a few hours.

Keywords Intensive care unit • Mechanical ventilation • Withdrawal of treatment Multi-organ failure • Liverpool care pathway

The intensive care unit (ICU) is a setting in which critically ill patients receive high-intensity treatments and procedures to sustain life and reverse disease processes [1]. The initial focus is driven by the need to prevent death using invasive technologies such as endotracheal mechanical ventilation, vasopressor agents, nasogastric nutrition, and multiorgan support (Fig. 12.1). This may seem to be at the opposite end of

A.D. Gascoigne, M.B.B.S., FRCP, B.Sc.
Department of Critical Care Medicine,
Royal Victoria Infirmary, Newcastle upon Tyne, UK

S.J. Bourke, M.D., FRCP, FRCPI, DCH (✉)
Department of Respiratory Medicine, Royal Victoria Infirmary,
Queen Victoria Road, Newcastle upon Tyne NE1 4LP, UK
e-mail: stephen.bourke@nuth.nhs.uk

S.J. Bourke, E.T. Peel (eds.), *Integrated Palliative Care of Respiratory Disease*,
DOI 10.1007/978-1-4471-2230-2_12, © Springer-Verlag London 2013

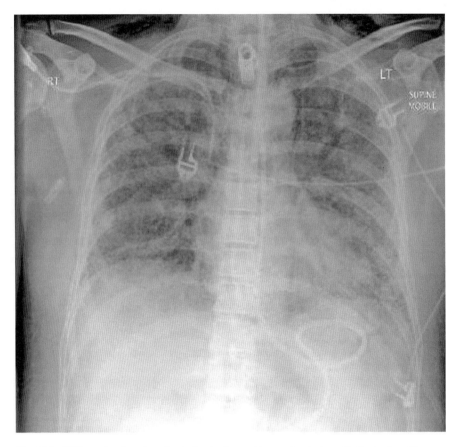

Fig. 12.1 ICU care involves invasive technologies such as mechanical ventilation and multi-organ support, with intensive physiological monitoring, to sustain life. These critically ill patients are at high risk of dying and palliative care is a crucial component of comprehensive ICU care

the spectrum of medical care from palliative medicine where the focus is often on relieving distress and suffering as life declines to a natural end. However, these critically ill patients are at high risk of dying such that ICU clinicians are involved in managing dying patients and their families on a daily basis, and the ethos, knowledge, and skills of palliative medicine are particularly important in this setting [2–4].

Furthermore, palliative care on ICU is not confined to dying patients. Patients who respond well to ICU care and who recover experience a high level of symptoms and distress during their critical illness and need skilled palliation and relief of suffering throughout their care [5–7]. Palliative care is therefore a crucial component of comprehensive ICU care and must run in parallel with high-intensity interventions at all stages of ICU management.

There are particular aspects of palliative care on ICU that need special consideration. In many cases, the critically ill patient is unable to communicate and discussions and decisions then often involve family members acting as surrogates for the patient [8, 9]. Particular skills are needed in managing complex clinician–family–patient communication in the context of catastrophic illness and a distraught family. Often the ICU team will not have known the patient previously. In patients who deteriorate progressively despite intensive treatment, the ICU team must exercise good clinical judgment in recognizing when such treatment is merely prolonging the dying phase rather than sustaining life. The focus of care then transitions from attempts at maintaining life to making the dying process as comfortable and dignified as possible. Because of the severity of the illness of these critically ill patients, the end of life phase is often short, typically lasting only a few hours [10, 11]. In the past there was criticism of the management of death and dying on ICUs but nowadays there is increasing evidence that ICU teams can provide excellent end of life care [5, 7]. A survey of the families of patients who died on ICU showed that the families generally felt that they had been well supported, that communication had been good, and that the patient had been kept comfortable when dying [7]. Most families felt that the patient's life had neither been prolonged nor shortened unnecessarily and that the patient and the family had been treated with respect and compassion. Although the clinical team will be experiencing regret at the failure of high-intensity care to reverse the disease process, they can find it professionally fulfilling to support patients and their families through the dying process. Satisfaction with end of life care is a key indicator of the quality of ICU care [3, 4].

Intensive Care of Respiratory Disease

Intensive care is a means of delivering a higher level of physiological monitoring, organ support, therapeutic intervention, and nursing care than can routinely be delivered on general wards [1]. Patients are acutely ill and have deteriorated, or are expected to deteriorate, as a consequence of their presenting illness. Without intensive interventions their recovery may be compromised and their risk of death significantly increased. In some cases, there is an acute severe illness, such as pneumonia, in a previously healthy patient [12]. Because of the severity of the illness, the patient is at high risk of dying but has the potential to recover with high-intensity care in the ICU. Under these circumstances, most patients will want to have ICU level care. In many cases, an acute crisis occurs in the course of chronic progressive lung disease. A patient with irresectable lung cancer may become acutely ill with a pulmonary embolism, major hemoptysis, or pneumonia [13]. The immediate problem is treatable, although life expectancy from the underlying cancer may be limited. Similarly a patient with cystic fibrosis or advanced bronchiectasis may suffer a major hemoptysis or pneumothorax causing an acute crisis [14]. Aspiration pneumonia may occur in a patient compromised by neuromuscular disease and chronic respiratory failure. Acute exacerbations occur in the course of many chronic lung diseases such as chronic obstructive pulmonary disease (COPD), cystic fibrosis, or fibrotic lung disease [8, 14–17]. The decision to admit the patient to ICU should be on the basis that the deterioration is due to a reversible or at least partially recoverable process. These are complex decisions for the patient, the family, and the clinical team and it can be difficult to incorporate such acute crises into advance care planning as patients who may wish to be at home if they are dying may also want to have intensive treatment if there is a reasonable prospect of recovery. In some cases, the deterioration is due to progression of the underlying disease and there may be no identifiable reversible cause. Thus the outcome for patients with idiopathic pulmonary fibrosis admitted to ICU for respiratory support is generally poor unless a reversible complication is present [16, 17].

There are several scoring systems used to try to predict which patients are unlikely to benefit from ICU level care, such as the APACHE score (acute physiology and chronic health evaluation). However, such scoring systems have substantial limitations and do not accurately predict the outcome in an individual patient [18]. Poor prognostic features include the absence of a reversible cause for the deterioration, diminished preceding functional reserve with impairment in activities of daily living, additional disease in other organ systems, and the development of multi-organ failure.

Decision to Admit to ICU

ICU care is inherently intrusive and burdensome, and some patients with advanced chronic lung disease may not wish to undergo ICU care, particularly if their deterioration is likely to indicate a progression of the underlying disease rather than a reversible complication. Failed ICU care under these circumstances may impose additional suffering and detract from the end of life experience of both the patients and their families [19]. Admission to ICU before death in the face of known poor prognosis may represent poor clinical judgment and decision making. Some studies raise concerns that patients being admitted to ICU may not have had comprehensive honest information about their prognosis and may not have had discussion of palliative care as an alternative [20]. Decisions to escalate to ICU level care often have to be made quickly and there is sometimes reluctance on the part of physicians to discuss the limitations of ICU care and the likely prognosis.

In some circumstances, it may be appropriate to set a "ceiling of care" whereby there is a trial of treatment and ICU support to reverse the disease process but with a recognition that if treatment fails or additional multi-organ complications occur ICU care should rapidly transition to focus on palliative end of life care. Ideally for many patients with chronic lung disease advanced care planning should have already addressed the patient's wishes. In practice the patient and family may find it difficult to decide in advance, particularly when an acute crisis changes the situation. Further discussions will be needed at the time of crisis. Discussion of prognosis and the patient's wishes and expectations are an important part of routine consultations in patients with progressive respiratory disease. Sometimes such discussions can be particularly complex, such as in the case of patients with advanced cystic fibrosis who may be close to death but hoping for a rescue lung transplantation [21]. Under these circumstances, palliative measures and some end of life discussions are still appropriate even where the disease trajectory may be dramatically altered by transplantation.

When a patient is admitted to hospital, early involvement of the ICU team may help in the discussion of the role and limitations of ICU care. There is a developing concept in ICU medicine of "care without walls" whereby the ICU setting is only part of a continuum of care for critically ill patients [1]. "Critical care outreach" involves the ICU team seeing patients on general wards and emergency departments so that there is early discussion of the role of ICU level care. The ICU team can support physicians in delivering care on medical wards and in deciding on the appropriateness of escalating care to the ICU setting. It should be recognized that high-intensity interventions are, of course, not confined to the ICU setting. Some patients with chronic respiratory failure receive long-term non-invasive ventilation at home. Patients with cystic fibrosis frequently receive high-intensity interventions at home including gastrostomy feeding and intravenous antibiotics administered via central venous access devices. Patients recovering from critical illness may be transferred from the ICU to "step down" care on a respiratory ward with post-ICU support from the "critical care outreach" team, particularly if the patient is receiving non-invasive ventilation or requires care of a tracheostomy. Patients and their families may be concerned at a change from a high level of staffing, such as one-to-one nursing, on the ICU to a lower level of staffing and support on a general ward. Many patients recovering from critical illness need ongoing rehabilitation, including psychological support, in recovering from the trauma of an acute illness. ICU follow-up clinics are being developed to manage the many long-term physical and psychological complications arising from critical illness, such as neuromyopathies, post-extubation airway problems, cognitive syndromes, and psychological problems, such as posttraumatic stress disorder.

There are substantial differences in how ICU level care is delivered in different countries and different hospitals [1]. It is increasingly recognized that intensive care is an applied principle and does not have boundaries and is not confined to the ICU setting [22]. When a patient's condition necessitates admission to the high-technology ICU environment, with care delivered by a specialist ICU team, this should not be to the exclusion of the parent team, who should continue to be involved with both the patient and the family, particularly where long-term relationships may have already been established.

Symptom Control on ICU

Critical illness is often associated with distressing symptoms such as pain, breathlessness, and anxiety [3–6]. The ICU setting is frightening for the patients and their families with high-technology equipment, noise from monitors, high levels of activity and bright lighting with some loss of day-night cycles. ICU interventions are inherently intrusive and burdensome. Nowadays ICU teams routinely include palliation of symptoms and distress in their overall care plan. It is important to be vigilant for specific symptoms such as pain, agitation, delirium, and distress [10, 11, 23]. Scoring systems, such as 10-point scales, may be used to quantify such symptoms and to assess the response to treatments with sedative and pain-relieving medications. Particular attention is needed with interventions that are known to cause distress and pain, such as endotracheal intubation, insertion of central venous or urinary catheters, insertion of nasogastric tubes and suctioning of the airway [24]. Other procedures, such as turning the patient in bed, have also been identified as causing particular distress. There are often difficulties in assessing symptoms in patients in ICU as many have an impaired level of consciousness and difficulties in communicating their needs when on mechanical ventilation with sedation [2–5]. Many studies show that these patients have distressing symptoms that may be underestimated by the clinical team. Sleep disturbance can lead to disorientation and delirium, and efforts should be made to provide some day-night cycle with reduced lighting and use of clocks to help to orientate the patient in time. Delirious patients often subsequently report having had delusions of being kidnapped and subjected to harm. Symptom control, relief of distress, explanation, and reassurance are of paramount importance throughout the whole process of ICU care [24].

Opioids are the main drugs used for relief of pain because of their powerful analgesic effect with additional beneficial sedative and anxiolytic effects [10, 11]. Benzodiazepines help to relieve agitation and have additional useful amnesic properties, but need to be used judiciously, as sedation can be associated with increased morbidity and mortality [25]. Frequent visits by the family are often helpful in reassuring the patient, and the family should be encouraged to inform the ICU staff if they observe anything that they perceive as discomfort in the patient.

Withholding and Withdrawing Treatments

When it is recognized that therapeutic options have been exhausted and that technological interventions are merely prolonging the dying process rather than promoting recovery, a decision is usually made to withdraw such measures [4, 8, 26, 27]. This involves a change in the direction and goals of care with a transition to a focus on relieving symptoms and distress, when recovery is no longer achievable. Ideally all medical decisions about admission to ICU, escalating care to invasive procedures and the subsequent withdrawal of failing treatments should be made by the patient, the family and the medical team jointly, basing these decisions on the patient's wishes and the physician's judgment and knowledge. In the setting of critical illness on ICU, the patients are often unable to participate in these decisions, but nonetheless they remain the key focus, and are protected by the ethical principles of autonomy, beneficence, and non-maleficence, with the clinical team and family acting in their best interests if they are incapacitated [8, 26]. Any expressed wishes or advanced directives by the patient are of key importance. Discussions with the family involve the key principles of palliative care and medical ethics including exploration of what the patient would have wanted, explanation of surrogate decision making, and affirmation of non-abandonment (holistic care continues but the focus is relief of symptoms and distress). It is crucial that the family understand that they are not being asked to make the decision to withdraw or withhold any treatment, as this is not their role or responsibility and may result in undue guilt or distress.

The principles and practice of withdrawing life-sustaining treatments have been extensively considered and are widely accepted throughout the world. Guidance has been provided by many authorities including the American Thoracic Society, the American College of Critical Care Medicine, and the General Medical Council in the United Kingdom [3, 4, 27]. There is recognition that death is a natural end to life and that continuing futile treatments and interventions in patients who are dying is not in their best interests. It is acknowledged that such decisions can be difficult and distressing. It is clearly established that patients with mental capacity have a legal right to refuse treatment even where refusal of recommended treatment may result in harm to themselves or their death [27]. Conversely the guidance indicates that where a patient wishes to have a treatment that, in the doctors considered view, is not clinically indicated, there is no ethical or legal obligation on the doctor to provide it [27]. Decisions about whether to withhold or withdraw a life-prolonging treatment are the responsibility of the senior clinician in charge of the patient's care, taking account of the views of the patient, or those close to the patient. The aim should be to resolve any disagreements and to achieve consensus between the patient's wishes and the medical team's decisions. In difficult situations, particularly where there is a lack of consensus, it is often helpful to seek a second opinion or to have the case reviewed by an ethics committee. In some rare situations, specialist legal advice may be required to ensure compliance with legal requirements [26, 27]. The General Medical Council also indicates the need to ensure that there is proper care for the dying patient. Clearly palliative care does not in any way imply stopping care of the patient, but rather continuation of intensive measures focused on relieving symptoms and distress.

End of Life Care on ICU

The majority of deaths that occur on ICU involve a phase of recognition that the patient is progressively deteriorating despite intensive treatment followed by the withholding or withdrawal of life-sustaining support [8, 10, 11]. The focus of care then changes from attempted cure to palliation of symptoms and distress in a dying patient. Once life support is withdrawn death usually follows within a short period of time such that the end of life phase often lasts only a few hours [10]. This reflects the severity of the disease in these critically ill patients.

End of life care should be managed on an individual basis depending on the precise needs and circumstances of each particular patient. Intrusive treatments may be continued if they are contributing to the patient's comfort or if withdrawal might cause distress that was difficult to relieve. However, the goals of treatment have now changed from attempted cure to relief of suffering. When it is established that the patient is dying, a decision is made that attempted cardiopulmonary resuscitation would be futile and inappropriate. Failed treatments are usually withdrawn, including antibiotics, vasopressor and inotropic drugs, renal replacement therapy, and clinically assisted nutrition.

Decisions to withdraw endotracheal mechanical ventilation are more complex and need careful consideration [3, 4, 10]. There is the possibility that withdrawing mechanical ventilation could result in the patient struggling to breathe, which might not be fully controlled by opiate and sedative medication. This is not likely to occur if the patient is unconscious as a result of their critical illness. In other circumstances, it may be possible to withdraw mechanical ventilation so as to allow patients to have some communication with their family. Transfer to non-invasive ventilation may be an option under these circumstances, allowing communication for a period of time without the patient struggling to breathe. Sometimes patients who are dying from profound hypotension and progressive renal failure, for example, may be sufficiently alert to indicate their discomfort from their endotracheal tube and may be attempting to pull it out. Withdrawing of mechanical ventilation, or other intrusive interventions, at this stage, is on the basis that they are not relieving symptoms or distress, or that the patient no longer wants them, rather than on the basis of any intent to hasten death [8, 27].

Titrating the dose of benzodiazepines and opioids to relieve pain, breathlessness, and anxiety can be complex in patients who are being withdrawn from life support [10, 11]. Muscle-relaxant drugs are discontinued as they are not helpful in control of symptoms in patients who have stopped mechanical ventilation and they may mask symptoms. Some surveys of ICU nurses report frustrations that symptom control is not always optimal in these patients [28]. Inexperienced clinicians may be reluctant to use adequate doses of these medications for fear of hastening death [11]. However, studies clearly show that there is no evidence that proper use of these drugs to control symptoms after the withdrawal of life support hastens death. Doses need to be adjusted according to many factors including the patients' previous exposure to opioids, their renal and hepatic function, their level of distress, and the response to treatment. It is important that ICU nurses and doctors should be vigilant and experienced in evaluating signs of distress in patients who cannot communicate, and that the dose of medication is titrated to ensure comfort. Use of the Liverpool Care Pathway for the dying patient can help ensure optimal end of life care for patients dying on ICUs [29]. Specialist palliative care teams can support ICU teams in providing holistic care for these patients.

Integrating Palliative Care into ICUs

ICU clinicians are frequently involved in managing dying patients and their families such that they have considerable knowledge and experience of palliative care in the ICU setting. It is clear that palliative care is a crucial component at all stages of

ICU care and that there are particular issues in end of life care in patients who have been receiving life support. The skills, knowledge, and ethos of palliative medicine are a core component of holistic ICU care and should be central to ICU training and educational programmes [3, 4]. Specialist palliative care teams can provide additional benefit to these patients, particularly in supporting ICU clinicians when discussing distressing information and decisions with families and when implementing the Liverpool Care Pathway for the dying patient [6, 9, 19]. In some cases, palliative care teams may have already been involved as part of the multidisciplinary care of patients with chronic lung disease. This is increasingly the case for patients with COPD, neuromuscular disease, cystic fibrosis, and progressive fibrotic lung disease where there is a move to involve palliative care teams earlier in the course of the disease to improve symptom control and to facilitate advance care planning, rather than to confine specialist palliative care input to the terminal stages of the disease. It may be helpful for a member of the specialist palliative care team to attend meetings with the family to provide additional practical and emotional support [2, 9]. A specialist palliative care consultation may be particularly helpful if families are not coping with the discussions or are experiencing anger, guilt, denial, or other complex emotions. This may particularly be the case if there is a lack of consensus about decisions, if there are particular concerns about common end of life issues such as nutrition and hydration, or if there is difficulty in controlling complex symptoms [2, 19, 27]. ICU teams are usually very experienced at making decisions about use and withdrawal of life-supporting treatments, and have considerable knowledge and experience of the use of opioids and sedatives in the ICU setting. Palliative care teams can provide expertise in additional areas such as meeting the religious and emotional needs of patients and families during the critical illness and in the bereavement phase [29]. The precise role of a specialist palliative care team will depend on the experience of the ICU team and the circumstances of practice in a particular hospital. Sometimes the palliative care team can facilitate the transfer of dying patients from the ICU to a general ward, or even to their home, if that is their wish [30].

Patient and family satisfaction with communication, symptom control, relief of distress, and end of life care are key outcome measures for ICUs, and there is increasing evidence that a very high level of palliative care can be achieved in this setting [7].

References

1. Vincent JL, Singer M. Critical care: advances and future perspectives. Lancet. 2010;376: 1354–61.
2. Bailly N, Perrier M, Bougle MF, Colombat C, Colombat P. The relationship between palliative and intensive care. Eur J Palliat Care. 2003;10:199–201.
3. Truog RD, Campbell ML, Curtis JR, et al. Recommendations for end-of-life care in the intensive care unit: a consensus statement by the American College of Critical Care Medicine. Crit Care Med. 2008;36:953–63.

4. Lanken PN, Terry PB, DeLisser HM, et al. An official American Thoracic Society clinical policy statement: palliative care for patients with respiratory diseases and critical illnesses. Am J Respir Crit Care Med. 2008;177:912–27.

5. Desbiens NA, Wu AW, Broste SK, et al. Pain and satisfaction with pain control in seriously ill hospitalized adults: findings from the SUPPORT research investigations. Crit Care Med. 1996;24:1953–61.

6. White DB, Luce JM. Palliative care in the intensive care unit: barriers, advances and unmet needs. Crit Care Clin. 2004;20:329–43.

7. Heyland DK, Rocker GM, O'Callaghan CJ, Dodek PM, Cook DJ. Dying in the ICU: perspectives of family members. Chest. 2003;124:329–97.

8. Simmonds AK. Ethics and decision making in end stage lung disease. Thorax. 2003;58: 272–7.

9. Curtis JR, Engelberg RA, Wenrich MD, Shannon SE, Treece PD, Rubenfeld GD. Missed opportunities during family conferences about end of life care in the intensive care unit. Am J Respir Crit Care Med. 2005;171:844–9.

10. Hall RI, Rocker GM. End of life care on ICU: treatments provided when life support was or was not withdrawn. Chest. 2000;118:1424–30.

11. Chan JD, Treece PD, Engelberg RA, et al. Narcotic and benzodiazepine use after withdrawal of life support: association with time of death? Chest. 2004;126:286–93.

12. Woodhead M, Welch CA, Harrison DA, Bellinghan G, Ayres JG. Community-acquired pneumonia on the intensive care unit: secondary analysis of 17869 cases in the ICNARC case mix programme database. Crit Care. 2006;10:1–9.

13. Toffart AC, Minet C, Raynard B, et al. Use of intensive care in patients with non-resectable lung cancer. Chest. 2011;139:101–8.

14. Sood N, Paradowski J, Yankaskas JR. Outcomes of intensive care unit care in adults with cystic fibrosis. Am J Respir Crit Care Med. 2001;163:335–8.

15. Wildman MJ, Harrison DA, Brady AR, Rowan K. Case mix and outcomes for admissions to UK adult, general critical care units with chronic obstructive pulmonary disease: a secondary analysis of the ICNARC case mix programme database. Crit Care. 2005;9:s38–48.

16. Xaubet A, Molina MM, Badia JR, Torres A. Outcome of patients with interstitial lung diseases requiring mechanical ventilation. Clin Pulm Med. 2005;12:26–31.

17. Blivet S, Philit F, Sab JM, et al. Outcome of patients with idiopathic pulmonary fibrosis admitted to the ICU for respiratory failure. Chest. 2001;120:209–12.

18. Barnato AE, Angus DC. Value and role of intensive care unit outcome prediction models in end of life decision making. Crit Care Med. 2004;20:345–62.

19. Shippey B, Winter B. End of life care. In: Nimmo GP, Singer M, editors. ABC of intensive care. London: Blackwell publishing Ltd; 2011. p. 71–3.

20. Rady MY, Johnson DJ. Admission to intensive care unit at the end of life: is it an informed decision. Palliat Med. 2004;18:705–11.

21. Bourke SJ, Doe SJ, Gascoigne AD, et al. An integrated model of provision of palliative care to patients with cystic fibrosis. Palliat Med. 2009;23:512–7.

22. Eddlestone J, Goldhill D, Morris J. Levels of critical care for adult patients. London: Intensive Care Society; 2009. http://www.ics.ac.uk/jics_publications/. Accessed Apr 2012.

23. Mularski RA. Pain management in the intensive care unit. Crit Care Clin. 2004;20:381–401.

24. Turner JS, Briggs SJ, Springhorn HE, Potgieter PD. Patients' recollection of intensive care unit experience. Crit Care Med. 1990;18:966–8.

25. Toft P, Strom T. Update on sedation and analgesia in mechanical ventilation. Eur Respir Mon. 2012;55:229–38.

26. Luce JM, Alpers A. Legal aspects of withholding and withdrawing life support from critically ill patients in the United States and providing palliative care to them. Am J Respir Crit Care Med. 2000;162:2029–32.

27. General Medical Council. Treatment and care towards the end of life: good practice in decision-making. London: GMC; 2010. http://www.gmc-uk.org/End_of_life/32486688.pdf. Accessed Apr 2012.

28. Ferrand E, Lemaire F, Regnier B, et al. Discrepancies between perceptions by physicians and nursing staff of intensive care unit end of life decisions. Am J Respir Crit Care Med. 2003;167:1310–5.
29. Chapman L. Adapting the Liverpool care pathway for intensive care units. Eur J Palliat Care. 2009;16:116–8.
30. Beuks BC, Nijhof AC, Meertens JH, Ligtenberg JJ, Tulleken JE, Zijlstra JG. A good death. Intensive Care Med. 2006;32:752–3.

Part IV
End-of-Life Care

Chapter 13
End of Life Care

Paul Paes and Eleanor Grogan

Abstract The term interstitial lung disease covers a number of conditions affecting the interstitium of the lung. The commonest of these is idiopathic pulmonary fibrosis (IPF). IPF usually presents with breathlessness and/or cough. The three pillars of care management strategy include (1) disease-centered management, (2) symptom-centered management, and (3) education and self-management. Sadly there is no strong evidence of any beneficial drug treatment on the natural history of IPF, although oxygen and lung transplant may both have a role. The symptomatic management of breathlessness and cough, as well as the other symptoms of more advanced disease, is considered in other chapters. The chapter concludes with a ten-point approach to the palliative management of IPF patients.

Keywords Idiopathic pulmonary fibrosis • Disease management • Symptom management Self management • Breathlessness • Cough

To cure sometimes, to relieve often, to comfort always (Anon. 16th century)

P. Paes, M.B.B.S., M.Sc., MMedEd, FRCP (✉)
Department of Palliative Care,
Northumbria Healthcare NHS Foundation Trust, Newcastle University,
North Shields, Tyne and Wear, UK

North Tyneside General Hospital,
Rake Lane, North Shields, Tyne and Wear NE29 8NH, UK
e-mail: paul.paes@nhct.nhs.uk

E. Grogan, B.Sc., M.B.B.S., M.A., FRCP
Department of Palliative Care, Wansbeck General Hospital,
Woodhorn Lane, Ashington, Northumberland NE63 9JJ, UK

S.J. Bourke, E.T. Peel (eds.), *Integrated Palliative Care of Respiratory Disease*,
DOI 10.1007/978-1-4471-2230-2_13, © Springer-Verlag London 2013

Introduction

The earlier chapters have looked at specific conditions and the major palliative care issues in each. In progressive respiratory conditions, the focus of care transitions from therapies directed against the disease to palliative management of the effects of the disease process. Often this realization can feel like a failure of medical treatment and cause clinicians and patients to feel a loss of hope. Palliative care is an approach that improves the quality of life of patients and their families facing the problems associated with life-threatening illness, through the prevention and relief of suffering by means of early identification and impeccable assessment and treatment of pain and other problems, physical, psychosocial, and spiritual [1]. In doing so, palliative care aims to give some control back to patients and clinicians by focusing on what can be done to improve the situation and acknowledging those areas which cannot be addressed.

This chapter addresses end of life care, incorporating thinking about both the last few days of life and the last year of life. The focus of the first part of the chapter is on identifying those patients who are likely to die in the next year, and planning their care appropriately. For these patients disease-modifying therapies, emergency treatments, palliative care, and supportive care must run in parallel. A framework of care across primary and secondary care is set out including key issues around communication, anticipatory planning, clinical decision making, and ethics. The second part of the chapter focuses on the last few days of life and practical steps in managing this stage.

Recognizing That a Patient Is Dying (or Is at Risk of Dying)

Recognizing that a patient is or may be approaching the end of life is a key skill for those involved in managing respiratory conditions. On a population level, it is relatively straightforward to estimate prognosis, based on the severity of a disease and other measurable factors. However, for individual patients, it is difficult to predict prognosis accurately in terms of time, and healthcare professionals are poor at doing this [2]. It can be especially difficult to determine whether an acute deterioration will be reversible or whether it may represent the onset of the dying phase.

There are a number of tools designed to help. In the UK, a national end of life strategy endorses the use of the gold standards framework which is designed to aid recognition of patients who are in the last 6–12 months of life, and provides a template for their care [3]. It suggests three triggers to identify patients in the last 12 months of life [4]:

1. To ask yourself "the surprise question": "Would you be surprised if this patient were to die in the next few months, weeks, or days?" This is an intuitive question, incorporating clinical assessment, knowledge, and experience.

2. General indicators of decline: deterioration, increasing need or patients who make the choice not to have further disease-modifying treatments.
3. Specific indicators relevant to the underlying condition.

Examples

Prognostic Indicator Guidance 2011 [4]

Cancer:

- Metastatic cancer
- Predictors for cancer patients are available, e.g., PiPS (UK validated Prognosis in Palliative care Study). Prognosis tools can help but should not be applied blindly.
- "The most important predictive factor in cancer is performance status and functional ability" – if patients are spending more than 50 % of their time in bed/lying down, prognosis is likely to be about 3 months or less.

Organ failure – erratic decline
Chronic obstructive pulmonary disease (COPD)

At least two of the indicators below:

- Disease assessed to be severe (e.g., FEV1 <30 % predicted)
- Recurrent hospital admissions (>3 in last 12 months)
- Fulfils long-term oxygen therapy criteria
- Medical Research Council dyspnea score 4/5 – breathless after 100 m on the level or confined to house
- Features of right heart failure
- Other factors, such as anorexia, admission to intensive care unit, or need for non-invasive ventilation.
- More than 6 weeks of systemic steroids in the preceding 6 months.

None of these triggers can accurately predict prognosis in an individual patient and they need to be used judiciously but they are aimed at identifying a group of patients who have advanced disease and are at risk of dying in the next 6–12 months, whilst acknowledging that they may well live longer. There are significant disparities between the levels of palliative care provided to patients with different diagnoses [5, 6]. This is partly due to the inherent unpredictability of some lung diseases. However, it is necessary to avoid "prognostic paralysis" which can prevent the patient from receiving appropriate supportive end of life care. If the needs of these patients can be identified sooner, discussion of the patient's wishes, anticipation of clinical problems, and patient-centered planning can be performed in a timely fashion rather than during a crisis.

Example
Mrs Smith is 75 years of age and she has a long history of COPD. She has been having increasingly frequent hospital admissions for treatment of exacerbations and she is clearly less well than she was 6 months ago.

Although her prognosis is uncertain, it would not be a surprise if she died in the next year. It would therefore be sensible to start having discussions about this with her. If she realizes that she may be approaching the end of her life, then she will have the opportunity to plan things such as writing a will, visiting people she wants to see, or doing particular things she would like to do before she dies. Recognizing that a patient may be at risk of dying in the next 6–12 months does not mean stopping disease-modifying treatment or changing the management plan, unless this is clinically indicated or due to patient preferences. Instead, it is about considering the measures that might be taken to improve quality of life now and in preparation for the dying stage.

Palliative Care Registers

It is now common in the UK for primary care physicians to have palliative care registers to aid planning the care of patients in this phase of their illness. These registers are evolving as a means of improving delivery of palliative care to patients with advanced disease. Placing patients on the palliative care register leads to the planning of their care as well as regular multi-professional discussions of their needs. Crucial to this are discussions with patients and their families at an appropriate pace and timing, recognizing that some patients may not want to address or discuss these issues.

Respiratory and palliative care teams play a crucial role in the identification and ongoing care of patients on palliative care registers. Informing primary care that a patient is appropriate to go on the palliative care register is a crucial step in highlighting their needs and it may also open up extra services and finances for patients and carers.

Example
Mr Brown is a 45-year-old man with a long history of smoking who presents to the emergency department in an emaciated state with hemoptysis. He is diagnosed after bronchoscopy and computed tomography as having metastatic non-small cell carcinoma of his lung. His WHO performance status is 2–3.

Mr Brown has a poor prognosis and meets the criteria for the palliative care register. This means that he will be regularly reviewed, to assess and manage any problems that arise, to plan for the future, and to provide support for his immediate family.

If he were to respond well to anti-cancer treatment, his name could be removed from the register.

The End of Life Pathway

Patients who are recognized as being in the palliative phase of their illness require careful discussion, assessment, and management of the situation and coordination of care, backed up by a range of support and specialist services [7] (Fig. 13.1).

Crucial to delivering good end of life care is the recognition that palliative care often runs in parallel with disease-modifying treatment and emergency care. This allows full medical treatment to continue whilst overcoming the current reality of respiratory patients often failing to have their palliative care needs addressed [8].

A number of issues need to be addressed for this group of patients and their families:

- Communication and information needs
- Patients' current clinical needs:
    Physical symptoms such as breathlessness or pain and psychological symptoms such as anxiety and depression
- Patients' future clinical needs:
    Anticipate and plan for problems as the condition deteriorates
- Current personal and social care needs
- Future personal and social care need

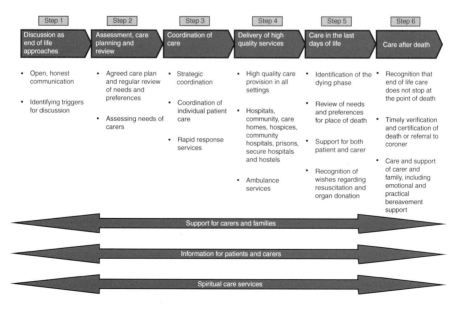

Fig. 13.1 Comprehensive end of life care

Communication

Good communication is the key to managing the end of life phase well. Patients and their families value honest and open communication. Many patients want to know more than they are currently being told and find healthcare professionals reluctant to talk about their issues [9–11]. A particular concern is a lack of understanding among patients of the severity and prognosis of progressive, non-malignant conditions such as COPD, fibrotic lung disease, and advanced bronchiectasis. A majority of complaints about end of life care are in relation to communication [12].

Clinicians often want to protect patients from losing hope, or worry that patients may not be ready for key discussions. Sometimes there is a reluctance to acknowledge treatment failure, uncertainty about prognosis, or a lack of time and skill to undertake such conversations. One of the goals of this book is to reinforce the concept that active disease-modifying care can run alongside palliative care, and that palliative care is not entirely dependent on an accurate prognosis. Patients often expect healthcare professionals to lead these conversations, and pick up on the professional reluctance to discuss them. Sometimes questions such as "How do you see the situation/future?" "What hopes/fears do you have?" or "What worries you most about the future?" can be useful triggers to such discussions.

Patients and families have mixed requirements for information, sometimes not having enough information and at other times being overloaded. A flexible approach is essential. Opportunities to discuss issues may need to be given repeatedly. Often the style of communication is as important as the words that are said. Key components include the following:

Exploring understanding

What do the patients know?
What are their expectations?
What do they want to know?
Do they want anyone else to be present?
Do they have particular concerns?
Do they have particular hopes or goals?

Dealing with difficult questions, such as about prognosis

Is the patient asking the question because they want an answer? Often patients are not after specific answers but want to discuss worries.
If time was short, would they want to know this? What difference would that information make and to whom?
If time was short, what would the patient want to do or say?
Where would they wish to be cared for and by whom?
What would help the situation now?

> **Example**
> Mrs Smith is 75 years of age and she has advanced progressive COPD. She is the main carer for her husband who is older. She has been having increasingly frequent hospital admissions for exacerbations and is less well than previously. She knows the situation is changing, and asks her doctor about his thoughts on her future.

In addressing this situation, understanding the motivation behind this question is important. Is she worried about the future, either for herself or her husband? Does she need to make specific plans? What would be helpful for her? Key aspects of communicating include listening as well as talking, recognizing uncertainty, and acknowledging anxiety and distress. Patients do not always expect answers, but appreciate an honest acknowledgement of the situation and affirmation that whatever happens they will not be abandoned. Uncertainty about prognosis should not stop discussion – focusing on specific issues and how to address them is often easier than trying to guess the timing of those issues. Communication should occur only at a pace that is appropriate for the individual patient rather than forcing conversations to fit a professional timetable or checklist.

Clinical Management: Adjusting the Focus of Care

As patients approach the end of their life, there needs to be a shift in the focus of their care so that treatments are aimed at maximizing quality of life rather than just extending life. This requires recognition from both the patient and the clinical team that the patient is toward the end of life. The shift required in focus of care will be different for each individual patient but there needs to be acceptance that the aim of treatment is no longer curative.

Mrs Smith with progressive COPD may be reaching the end stages of her illness. She may have practical or emotional things she wishes to plan for. She may also want to think about how future exacerbations will be managed. She may consider whether she would rather spend time in hospital in the hope of prolonging life, or whether she would rather stay at home and accept that life may be shorter without some treatments. Depending on her precise clinical status, the medical team may strongly advocate hospital treatment or conversely may feel that further treatments are unlikely to help the situation. Decisions do not need to be made in one consultation. This should be an ongoing process. Sometimes it is appropriate to continue with intensive disease-modifying treatment because this can often be a way to relieve symptoms and to maximize quality of life.

Clinical Management: To Treat or Not to Treat

In patients with advanced disease, decisions have to be made about the appropriate level of treatment. Sometimes this decision is obvious. If a patient presents who is known to have very advanced disease which has now progressed such that the patient is dying, the benefit of burdensome treatments should be questioned. The treating clinician should always identify the intended benefit of the proposed treatment. Patients can be offered treatment to make them *feel* better, but this is not the same as making the underlying condition better. Conversely, patients may have advanced disease but present with an acute complication, such as a pneumothorax, that is reversible, and treatment is likely to relieve distress and may restore the previous quality of life.

Many respiratory diseases, such as COPD, cystic fibrosis, or fibrotic lung disease, follow a chronic disease trajectory, characterized by exacerbations and recovery against a background of slow progressive decline. It is possible that one of these exacerbations may be the last one and that the patient may not recover but it can be difficult to tell when this will occur. This is very different from a typical cancer trajectory. Models of palliative care provision which make an artificial divide between disease-modifying treatment and palliative care are usually inappropriate for patients with chronic lung disease. Palliative care providing symptom relief and support needs to run in parallel with disease-modifying treatments and emergency care for acute exacerbations and complications. When it is uncertain whether a deterioration is reversible or not, it is reasonable to offer a trial of treatment, and patients may have clear wishes about how they wish to be treated. Treatment options should be explained, including the option of comfort measures only. If a trial of treatment, such as non-invasive ventilation, is being considered, it may be appropriate to discuss the concept of a ceiling of care.

> **Example**
> Mrs Smith has advanced progressive COPD. She has been struggling to manage at home for several weeks and is now spending much of her day asleep in bed. She presents unwell with another exacerbation. On previous admissions she has made it clear that she does not like being in hospital and is getting tired of life.

Mrs Smith needs a frank and honest discussion about her understanding of her disease and the treatment options, including the option of no treatment. Because exacerbations make her severely unwell and breathless, she is keen to try treatments but says that if it is clear that they are not working, then she would like her symptoms managed in alternative ways. She has always made it clear that she would like to die in her own home.

Having a frank and honest discussion, including acknowledging the possibility that treatment may not work and she may die, may allow her to express her preferences about end of life care – both what she would want and where she would want it.

CPR or DNACPR

In such circumstances, it is also appropriate to consider whether cardiopulmonary resuscitation (CPR) would be appropriate in the event of a cardio-respiratory arrest. This is an area that is emotive as, if not well handled, patients and their relatives may feel that they have been unfairly denied a treatment. Terminology is changing from DNAR (Do Not Attempt Resuscitation) to DNACPR (Do Not Attempt Cardiopulmonary Resuscitation) as this order specifically relates to the one treatment (CPR) and not other forms of treatments and resuscitation, such as fluid resuscitation. Current guidance in the UK comes from a joint statement by the British Medical Association, the Resuscitation Council and the Royal College of Nursing [13]. If no CPR decision has been made and the patient's wishes are unknown, the presumption should be in favor of CPR. The exception to this is in patients in whom attempting CPR would be clearly inappropriate; for example, a patient in the final stages of a terminal illness where death is imminent and unavoidable but for whom no formal DNAR decision has been made. CPR under these circumstances is not a realistic treatment option for the patient's condition, and is both futile and inappropriate. If it is felt that CPR would not re-start the patient's heart and breathing, then CPR should not be attempted. A patient does not have to be informed of a decision not to attempt CPR but should be informed of the severity of their condition. A more useful discussion may focus on the severity of their illness, the fact that they may be approaching the end of their life and that you would not do anything to unduly prolong this. However, any further questions the patient may have should be answered honestly and compassionately.

As with all treatments, there is likely to be a large group of patients in the middle where the likelihood of CPR working is unknown. If it is possibly a treatment that may benefit the patient, but you are not sure that this is the case, you may wish to discuss it with the patient to ascertain their wishes. This does not have to be phrased "do you want to be resuscitated if your heart stops?" but rather should be a discussion about their expectations of their condition and what they would want should anything happen unexpectedly. If the patient is deteriorating progressively and is in the dying phase of the disease, then CPR is not likely to be a feasible treatment and should not be offered as an illusory option.

Anticipatory Planning

One of the key reasons to identify that a patient is reaching the end phase of their illness is that it enables us to plan ahead and to deliver care that is consistent with a patient's wishes. Key to this is addressing current problems, but perhaps greater skill is required by the healthcare team to anticipate and plan for future problems. Decision making in this situation takes a number of forms and must comply with the legal and ethical frameworks of individual countries:

- Patient-driven decision-making tools: Advance Care Planning (ACP)
- Professionally driven decision making: Clinical Management Plans, emergency healthcare plans, treatment escalation plans.

Although these can be patient or professionally driven, they work best when done in partnership.

Advance Care Planning

Advance Care Planning is a voluntary process by which patients discuss their future wishes [14]. This is done in the anticipation of a future deterioration in a person's condition in case they lose the capacity to make those decisions as they arise. Many patients welcome this discussion, but others will not wish to participate. In the UK, the Mental Capacity Act indicates some legal options which patients can take:

Advance Decision to Refuse Treatment (ADRT) – this is a decision to refuse specific treatments. Set out correctly, this is legally binding. Common treatments refused include resuscitation, ventilation, feeding tubes, intravenous fluids, and antibiotics [15].

Lasting Power of Attorney – a patient may appoint someone to make decisions on their behalf in the future. This may be about healthcare issues or more financially based ones.

In addition to the legal options, many patients prefer a less formal approach. Some will be happy simply to discuss what is likely to happen, think about the future and their choices, but not wish to do anything more. Others will prefer to record some of those preferences in the form of an Advance Care Planning document or Advance Statement.

Advance Statement – This is a statement reflecting an individual's preferences and aspirations. It can help health professionals identify how the person would like to be treated and record past, present, and future wishes. It is the documented result of an Advance Care Planning discussion. Crucially it is not legally binding, which means that healthcare professionals need to use their judgment in applying the values in the document to their decision making. For patients, this fact overcomes a fear that they may commit themselves to a decision which they may later regret. A powerful aspect of an Advance Statement is that it enables views to be communicated, checked, clarified, and then shared with others.

The sorts of issues that patients might include in an Advance Care Planning discussion are:

- The patient's preferred place of care during the duration of their life
- Where they would like to be if they are dying
- General care preferences
- How active treatment should be if a complication develops
- Decisions about swallowing: nutrition and hydration
- Resuscitation status
- Management of incontinence
- Organ donation and
- Any other areas of importance

When a patient's condition deteriorates, the loss of control experienced can be overwhelming. Involving them in decision making restores some control over events. Literature in this area suggests that respiratory patients seldom get the chance to have these discussions before emergency situations arise and that they would welcome such discussions [16]. It is important to recognize that Advance Care Planning decisions only apply if a patient loses capacity. While a patient has capacity they should be consulted. Equally patients change their minds, and care should be taken in interpreting plans and updating them. Useful training modules on Advance Care Planning are included on the e-learning End of Life Care website [17].

Professionally Driven Decision Making

Advance Care Planning is a voluntary process that is dependent on patients wishing to plan for anticipated changes in their condition. Whether that takes place or not, healthcare professionals need to have clear management plans, which anticipate and address potential problems.

Clinical Management/Care Plans

The most straightforward option is to simply have a management plan agreed between primary care, secondary care, and the patient to address some of the following:

- What are the most likely clinical problems? Often these will be about exacerbations of the underlying respiratory condition, symptoms such as breathlessness and potential acute events such as infections or thrombo-embolic disease.

- What is the best management of these problems? What clinical signs should people look out for? What treatment works for this individual patient? What is the appropriate ceiling of care? What can be managed at home and when should an admission to hospital be considered?

A number of specific tools are emerging to aid this process:

- Emergency Healthcare Plans

    These documents are designed to give a specific plan to address an anticipated clinical problem where the right treatment is required promptly. Such a form is currently being introduced in the north east of England [18]. These plans are very specific to individuals.

- Treatment Escalation Plans

    These documents are designed to be used for patients who are deteriorating and for whom acute problems are anticipated. As a patient's health deteriorates, their ability to benefit from specific treatments lessens. Treatment escalation planning looks at specific treatments and considers whether a patient is likely to benefit. Importantly this needs to be an evolving document as a patient's situation changes. An example of a form used in Devon, UK, can be found in the reference quoted [19].

An Emergency Healthcare Plan is likely to be useful in managing a specific anticipated problem with a treatment plan. A Treatment Escalation Plan may be more helpful where a number of potential problems may arise, and guidance is required as to which specific treatments may be of benefit to a patient. Importantly clinical management plans, Emergency Healthcare Plans and Treatment Escalation Plans, are advisory plans and should guide clinical assessment and judgment, rather than replacing it. All of these approaches should include patients where possible in joint decision making and be consistent with any Advance Care Planning discussions.

Example

In our two case examples, Mr Brown has metastatic non-small cell carcinoma of his lung, and Mrs Smith has progressive COPD. Both are keen to talk about the future – Mr Brown has very clear views about how he wants his health managed. Mrs Smith feels she would like her doctors to make decisions for her as she does not feel her knowledge of treatments is good enough to make clear decisions.

Both patients would benefit from Advance Care Planning discussions. Both may benefit from making Advance Statements if they have particular preferences. If Mr Brown wishes to make clear decisions to refuse certain treatments, an ADRT form may be helpful. This ADRT may cover most clinical scenarios if well written, but cannot ask for specific treatments. Both patients would benefit from clear clinical care planning. In particular, Mrs Smith with her frequent exacerbations would benefit from the medical team considering how further exacerbations should be managed. Treatment escalation planning, an emergency healthcare plan, or simply a clinical management plan may all be helpful in managing an acute deterioration.

Ethics

Withholding, Withdrawing and Futile Treatments

Sometimes deciding whether or not to start a treatment can be difficult, especially in a patient with a respiratory illness when their disease trajectory may be difficult to predict. It may feel more comfortable to not start a treatment than to start one and then stop it, but there are many ethical issues to consider in this area.

> **Example**
> Mr Brown is a 45-year-old man with metastatic non-small cell carcinoma of his lung. His WHO performance status is 2–3.

Although Mr Brown has a new diagnosis of lung cancer and is relatively young, he has a poor performance status and it is uncertain if he will tolerate or benefit from palliative chemotherapy. Is it ethically better to start chemotherapy and then stop it, or not start it at all?

The decision should remain a clinical one, rather than be influenced by his young age or emotions about withholding a treatment. If he meets the standard criteria to receive chemotherapy, then it should be offered to him. As with all patients he should have the intended benefits explained to him, alongside likely adverse effects and alternative options (including the option of no chemotherapy). It should be made clear that the treatment is with palliative, rather than curative, intent. If he so wishes, the treatment should be started and his response to treatment gauged. If it is clear that chemotherapy is providing no benefit, that the adverse effects outweigh any benefits or that his cancer is progressing despite the treatment, then it would be appropriate to stop treatment. The alternative would be to withhold chemotherapy from Mr Brown. This would mean not offering him the option of chemotherapy, rather than him declining the treatment. To do so would be to deny him the chance of a treatment that may prolong his life and reduce his symptoms. If he is clinically well enough to receive it and meets the relevant criteria, then he should be offered chemotherapy rather than not being offered it because of an incorrect moral feeling of stopping a treatment being harder than never having started it.

The situation would be different if he was clearly within the last few days or weeks of life. In these circumstances, chemotherapy is unlikely to provide any benefit but instead give him the burden of adverse effects. This may prevent him from doing things he needs to do and seeing people he wants to see before he dies. In this situation it would be appropriate to withhold chemotherapy, but it would be being withheld because this is the appropriate clinical decision rather than Mr Brown being denied a potentially beneficial treatment

Doctrine of Double Effect

A concern that is sometimes raised in the management of patients with advanced disease is that use of medications such as opioids or benzodiazepines might hasten death, although the intention is to alleviate symptoms. The doctrine of double effect is an ethical term that is sometimes used where the intention of treatment is good (symptom control), but the treatment may have foreseeable but unintended consequences (death). This is generally not a principle that is useful in clinical practice. The same level of rigor should be applied to the use of opioids and benzodiazepines as with drugs such as insulin. Insulin has the potential to cause harm if used inappropriately but the doctrine of double effect would never be used to defend such practice. In a similar way it should not be used to defend inappropriate use of symptom control medication. Symptom control medication should be gradually titrated upward from small doses. A dose of opioids or benzodiazepines should never be so big as to affect the patient's respiratory function. Pain (even when treated) remains a respiratory stimulus and antagonizes opioid-induced respiratory depression [20]. If a dose is given that is large enough to affect the patient's respiratory function, it does not suggest that the doctrine of double effect is required to justify the prescriber's actions. Rather it suggests that the dose is inappropriate [21].

Psychological and Spiritual Issues

Healthcare professionals generally have a reasonable understanding of psychological issues, and the role that thoughts have on a person's wellbeing. Emotional reactions tend to peak at key points such as at the time of diagnosis of a serious illness, when the disease progresses and when an acute crisis occurs. It is important to distinguish between normal reactions to stress and more persistent signs of adjustment disorders, anxiety, or depression. Many patients with chronic lung disease suffer greater psychological morbidity than those with cancer [12, 22]. Interventions range from supportive listening to psychological treatments such as cognitive behavioral therapy and medications such as anti-depressants and anxiolytics.

Spiritual issues are harder to define, but relate to a person's values and their search for meaning or purpose. The European Association for Palliative Care defines spirituality as: "The dynamic dimension of human life that relates to the way persons (individual and community) experience, express and/or seek meaning, purpose and transcendence, and the way they connect to the moment, self, to others, to nature, to the significant and/ or the sacred" [23]. Spiritual domains may be the key component in bringing together the physical, psychological, and social issues of a patient. Toward the end of life, many people start to review their life and seek:

- Affirmation and acceptance of their life, choices, and decisions
- Forgiveness and reconciliation of areas of their life where they feel they have unresolved issues
- Discovery of meaning and direction

Indicators of spiritual distress include:

- Sense of hopelessness, meaninglessness, powerlessness, becoming withdrawn, or having suicidal thoughts
- Intense suffering: Can't endure anymore, what's the point in going on? Loneliness, isolation, vulnerability
- Change in beliefs, loss of faith/culture, anger toward God, church, etc.
- Sense of guilt or shame: being punished, deserving to be ill
- Unresolved feelings about death, worries about going to sleep, the dark, etc.

> **Example**
> Mr Brown is a 45-year-old man with metastatic non-small cell carcinoma of his lung. His symptoms of breathlessness and pain have previously been well controlled. Recently his pain has been unbearable and the team feel he has been responding differently to them.

The expression of physical symptoms should not be attributed to non-physical causes without good reason, and in most situations the interaction between physical and spiritual is complex. However, intense suffering and changes in the way people behave are often warning signs. Without addressing spiritual issues, physical symptoms can sometimes be difficult to treat. In Mr Brown's case, during a hospital admission one of the healthcare assistants finds him crying in the bath. He has two young children and having been told there is nothing that can control the cancer, the reality is dawning on him that time is very short with them. The thought of not being there for his children is unbearable, but he also wants to prepare them for his death. He distances himself from them gradually, so that they turn more to his wife and others. It has been over this time that his pain has got much worse, and when he talks it is obvious that although the distancing plan was well intentioned, it is causing him great distress. His family are the driving force in his life, and emotionally he cannot just close down that side of his life, without it leaving a profound gap. Bringing these issues out into the open makes the problem more explicit, even if there may be no easy solution.

A skill in addressing spiritual and emotional issues is to recognize that we should avoid giving specific answers – some questions about life have no answer. People need to find their own answers. Sometimes sharing uncertainty can be more powerful than providing inappropriate answers. Religion may form a key component of a person's spiritual being.

Identifying the Last Days of Life

Identifying the dying phase can be difficult. Some respiratory conditions such as lung cancer, fibrotic lung disease, and neuromuscular conditions may follow more predictable trajectories. Conditions such as COPD and cystic fibrosis are inherently more difficult as the disease trajectory is characterized by exacerbations and remissions.

Pragmatic criteria for recognizing the last days of life include the patient:

- Having a terminal diagnosis and reaching the end of their anticipated life expectancy
- Having progressively deteriorated
- Becoming weaker, more dependent, and bedbound
- Becoming drowsier and having difficulty concentrating
- Having difficulty swallowing food or medication, with reduced oral intake
- Having no reversible cause of the deterioration, the treatment of a potentially reversible cause would be futile, or they do not want treatment

The last point is crucial. Where there is doubt about whether deterioration is reversible, active treatment is appropriate but care needs to be taken in the communication with patients and family members so that they are clear about the potential outcomes. Treatment needs to be carefully monitored so that there is a regular review until it is clear whether the patient is likely to survive this episode, or deteriorate and die.

The decision that a patient is dying can sometimes be incorrect. In a patient who is thought to be dying, an open mind should be kept and decisions reviewed. In the UK, newer models of care such as the AMBER (Assessment, Management, Best Practice, Engagement of patients and carers, for patients whose Recovery is uncertain) care bundle recognize the difficulty of this aspect of decision making [24]. The principle of AMBER is pragmatic and potentially very useful for respiratory patients in recognizing that many patients require disease-modifying treatments until near the end of life. However, these patients and their families also need good symptom control, psychological care, and communication of the severity of the situation.

Example
Mrs Smith has progressive COPD. She has been struggling to manage at home for several weeks and spending much of her day asleep in bed. On previous admissions she has made it clear that she does not like being in hospital and is getting tired of life. She presents unwell in respiratory failure with a further exacerbation.

Mrs Smith now needs a further discussion about her treatment options, including the option of no treatment. As she feels so unwell with shortness of breath and cough, she is keen to try antibiotics and non-invasive ventilation but says that if it is clear that they are not working she would like her symptoms managed in alternative ways. She has always made it clear that she would like to die in her own home. To achieve Mrs Smith's wishes requires a dual approach of active medical treatment of the exacerbation of her COPD but also acknowledgement that she may die during this episode. A trial of treatment is usually the most appropriate option. If treatment fails, a decision needs to be taken so that if she wants to die at home, this can be achieved.

Failure to recognize the last days of life may lead to the patient (and family):

- Being unaware that death is imminent
- Losing trust in the clinical team as the condition clearly deteriorates without any acknowledgement of this
- Getting conflicting messages from the team
- Being more likely to die with uncontrolled symptoms and less likely to be in place of choice
- Having inappropriate cardiopulmonary resuscitation at death
- Not having their psychological, cultural, and spiritual needs met
- Having complex bereavement problems

When it is clear that a patient is dying, discussion and decisions need to be made about how this process will be managed:

- Where does the patient/family want to be, and what is possible? For those patients who want to be at home, it should be possible to organize care to meet their needs. Others may prefer the safety of an inpatient or care home environment
- Making clear decisions about ceilings of care; resuscitation, fluids, antibiotics, stopping routine observations, investigations, etc.
- Addressing symptom, psychological and spiritual needs
- Communicating with other healthcare professionals to let them know what is happening

Liverpool Care Pathway for the Dying

The Liverpool Care Pathway (LCP) has been endorsed nationally in the UK as a tool to help deliver good quality end of life care. It acts as a prompt and checklist for ensuring that the needs of patients are met once a team has decided that the patient is dying [25]. It covers a range of domains across physical, psychological, spiritual, and communication issues. All of these areas need to be addressed. The LCP supports this process and has a number of checks in place to make sure dying patients are well cared for. Successful use of the LCP is dependent on staff being trained appropriately and applying it sensitively. Deciding that a person is dying requires team agreement and a patient should only be started on the LCP when the team are as certain as they can be. Sometimes we get this decision wrong – the LCP requires regular review to make sure that this decision remains under review and that those who are not dying are not mis-managed. The LCP is regularly updated to take into account developments in end of life care and decision making [26].

Place of Care

Figures for where patients would prefer to die in the UK are quoted as being approximately: at home 60 %, in hospital 15 %, in a hospice 15 %, and in a care home 0 %. These figures need be treated with some caution because studies in this area have looked at patients who have incurable conditions but prior to them experiencing the dying phase. As patients approach death, their preference for being at home drops significantly and the preference for a hospice type environment increases to about 40 % [27]. Patients with respiratory disease have the highest rate of dying in hospitals (69 %) and the lowest rate of dying in their own home (13 %) compared to other conditions [28]. The data indicate that more patients would like to die at home than currently do so. There is now a drive to improve end of life care services in the community. This should not be at the expense of end of life services in hospital where a large proportion of patients will continue to die. In most areas, there are teams based in the community to deliver care at the end of life and to facilitate rapid transfer of patients from hospital to their home when dying. The earlier this is planned, the less the likelihood of delays due to issues such as waiting for oxygen or equipment.

Keeping people at home depends on:

- Having services/equipment in place
- Making clear clinical decisions: What could go wrong? What problems could lead to a hospital admission? How would we manage deteriorations? What is the ceiling of care?
- Appropriately skilled healthcare professionals who can assess and manage unexpected situations 24 h a day

For other patients, either their clinical situation or preference leads to an inpatient admission, either to a palliative care setting or hospital ward. Many respiratory patients have longstanding relationships with their specialist care teams and may want their end of life care to be delivered on a respiratory ward. Ensuring there are appropriate facilities for dying patients and their families continues to be an important aspect of hospital care.

Clinical Decision Making

When a patient is dying, problems should be anticipated and planned for in accordance with the patient's wishes. As well as anticipating symptoms, healthcare professionals should anticipate acute changes. Patients who are actively dying may experience a cardiac arrest. Attempts at cardiopulmonary resuscitation are unlikely to be successful, but likely to be started if an active "Do Not Attempt Resuscitation" order has not been made. Plans should be made to deal with possible problems such as infection, bleeding, falls, or acute symptoms. Although the goals of management are comfort care, often the most effective way of dealing with symptoms is to address the underlying cause. Where more burdensome treatments are used, their effectiveness should be closely monitored and the treatment withdrawn if it is not effective. Involving the patient in decision making is crucial. Certain treatments such as intravenous antibiotics, being for active resuscitation and consideration of ventilation (even if limited to non-invasive ventilation) are likely to require a hospital admission. For patients who wish to stay at home, an active decision needs to be taken about withholding these treatments and managing the problem in a different way.

Physical Care

Routine observations and investigations should stop unless they support patient comfort. Active assessment and management of symptoms and care issues need to continue. This includes assessing the cause of any symptoms.

When a patient is dying, swallowing and absorption of drugs becomes problematic. Drugs are given parenterally, usually subcutaneously for comfort (or intravenously if people have long-term intravenous access that is being used). Medication is given on an as-required basis, unless the patient is already taking the medication regularly. If a patient requires a drug more than once a day or has been on a regular oral dose, the drug should usually be prescribed on a regular basis using a continuous syringe driver.

There may be specific drugs used for respiratory conditions, such as oxygen or nebulized bronchodilators, that continue to provide symptom relief. In addition, there needs to be anticipation of potential problems that may arise. Management of these problems tends to rely on medication as people become less able to manage non-pharmacological treatments. Common symptoms in the last days of life include:

Pain

- Morphine or diamorphine are usually the most appropriate strong opioids to manage most pains at this stage.
- Patients who have not previously had pain often get pain in the last days of life from musculoskeletal causes. Other analgesic options include rectal paracetamol, rectal, or injectable non-steroidal anti-inflammatory drugs.

Nausea

- The same problems that lead to agitation often lead to a chemical nausea.
- Cyclizine, haloperidol, or levomepromazine are commonly used.

Agitation

- Agitation is common and can be associated with confusion. Causes are multifactorial, including biochemical abnormalities, infection, and hypoxia.
- Benzodiazepines such as midazolam and antipsychotics such as haloperidol or levomepromazine can be helpful, as well as maintaining a calm environment and reassurance.

Breathlessness

- Strong opioids such as morphine or diamorphine reduce the perception of breathlessness.
- Benzodiazepines such as midazolam relieve anxiety associated with breathlessness.

Respiratory Secretions "Death Rattle"

- These build up when a patient is no longer able to clear normal respiratory tract secretions.
- The noise produced can be distressing to relatives, although patients are not usually affected. Sometimes an explanation and reassurance are enough.
- Positioning of the patient in a semi-prone state allows postural drainage.
- Anticholinergic drugs such as hyoscine hydrobromide, hyoscine butylbromide, or glycopyrronium are used to reduce secretions.

Appendix, at the end of the book, contains recommended starting doses of common drugs used at the end of life, and conversions of commonly used opioids to parenteral preparations. These drugs need to be titrated according to effect. Please note these are guidelines and advice should be taken for individual patients.

Other key components of physical care include bladder and bowel care, reviewing nutrition and hydration, mouth care, and skin and hygiene needs.

Nutrition and Hydration

Loss of interest in food and drink and a reduction in the need for food and fluids are features of somebody who is naturally dying. Patients should be supported to eat and drink naturally for as long as they are able to and wish to. Artificial fluids may be beneficial if a patient is experiencing uncontrolled thirst or symptoms due to dehydration. However, thirst can be due to other causes and therefore effectively managed in other ways – good mouth care (keeping the mouth clean, moist and free of infections such as thrush), adjusting the temperature of the room, and avoiding situations which exacerbate thirst such as high blood glucose levels. Clinically assisted nutrition, such as nasogastric tube feeding, may be indicated for those who are experiencing uncontrolled hunger but this is very rare in dying patients. In the last days of life, the goal of treatments is comfort. Giving too much fluid or nutrition may induce symptoms as the body struggles to cope with large volumes. Vomiting and bowel disturbances or fluid retention and excess respiratory secretions can be problems in these patients.

Families and healthcare professionals may be concerned that the patient is dying because of lack of hydration or nutrition, rather than the underlying disease process. It is important to establish that patients are dying from an underlying disease, and that eating and drinking less is a symptom of this process, rather than the cause. Care should be particularly taken where the patient appears to stabilize or improve; or where the process of actively dying takes longer than expected. If there is doubt, decision making should err toward preserving life and considering the use of fluids and nutrition. A second opinion may be helpful if there is disagreement over these decisions.

Psychological and Spiritual Care

Crucial to exploring these areas is making sure that a patient's language and communication abilities have been maximized. This may need the addition of equipment or a translator. Exploring the patient's understanding, their concerns, hopes, coping strategies, fears, feelings, beliefs, and values are crucial to good end of life care. Often unresolved apparent physical symptoms are due to non-physical problems that have not been addressed. Most issues can be dealt with by the clinical team trusted by the patient. There may be times when specialist input from psychology, chaplaincy, or palliative care is indicated, but for most patients being listened to by a person they trust is the key. The importance of simply being there, rather than always needing to do something, should not be underestimated. Patients appreciate not being abandoned, even if the healthcare professional does not always feel they are achieving something.

Exactly the same issues face families and informal carers. Care needs to be taken to ensure that consent has been given by the patient to talk about health details. However, caring for those around the dying patient becomes increasingly the goal of end of life care as death approaches.

Communication

The emotional and communication needs of patients and families increase as patients approach the end of their life. The quality of care and symptom burden that patients face will have a marked impact on the experience relatives have, and their subsequent bereavement. At the very end of life communication needs can evolve rapidly.

Clinical teams need to adapt quickly and to offer regular opportunities to discuss issues, but in a way that is subtle and avoids being intrusive. Family members require communication to be as clear and unambiguous as possible. In addition, they need to be able to access healthcare professionals readily, especially if they are at home. Communication between clinical teams is essential so that care is coordinated.

Care After Death

As well as ensuring that the patient's care before death is well planned and appropriate, it is also important to ensure that this continues after the patient's death. There may be discussions that can be had prior to the patient's death so that both the patient and their family know what to expect.

Verification of Death

The death of the patient needs to be verified by someone qualified to do this. Traditionally this was a doctor, but in the UK this role has now been extended to nurses (with suitable training). The person verifying the death need not have met the patient when they were alive.

Certification

In the UK, a death certificate must be issued before the death can be registered and funeral proceedings commence. This needs to be issued by a doctor who has previously met the patient and seen them alive within the last 2 weeks. If a patient dies at home this may pose difficulties. If the general practice team knows that the patient is dying and has been notified by the hospital that the patient is being transferred home for end of life care, they are able to visit that patient, to attend to the patient's needs, but also to ensure that a death certificate could be provided without undue complication. If a patient dies without being seen by a doctor in the preceding 2 weeks, in England they must be referred to the coroner.

Post-Mortem Examinations and Coroner Referrals

If a patient dies of a possible occupationally acquired illness, the death must be referred to the coroner and a post-mortem is likely to be undertaken. In other situations, a hospital post-mortem may provide helpful information. It is helpful to make families aware of these issues as early as possible, before death if appropriate.

Practical Tasks

After a patient dies there are many practical tasks for the family to remember to do. The death certificate must be obtained and the death registered with the registrar. The funeral must be organized – often patients who know that they are dying have specified some wishes that they want incorporating into the funeral. Health- and social-care professionals involved in the patient's care must be notified and any equipment in the house returned. UK agencies such as the Department for Work and Pensions (DWP) must be notified so that pensions and benefits are appropriately dealt with. Because there is so much to remember at such a difficult time in life, booklets are available to guide the family through the process: "What to do after a death in England and Wales" and "What to do after a death in Scotland" [29, 30].

Bereavement

Grief is natural and to be expected in bereavement. It may present in different ways. Some people feel numb, shocked, and unable to function normally. Others need to carry on with normal activities to try to maintain a structure to their life. There is no right or wrong way to experience grief, and it should be recognized as an individual process.

When a patient has a life-limiting illness, the bereavement process may start prior to their death as the family start thinking about the future. They may wish to plan things to help future memories and the grieving process, and this should be encouraged. This may include activities, seeing loved ones or developing memory boxes. Memory boxes are a way for the patient to collect memories to pass to another member of the family, for example, cards or items of special personal importance.

Grief persists for a long time after the patient dies and should not be expected to resolve quickly. Factors that influence the grief reaction include circumstances leading up to the patient's death, meaning of the relationship with the deceased, personal vulnerability and availability of social support [31]. Most individuals are resilient and can cope with bereavement without professional intervention. Evidence suggests that bereavement counseling only makes a difference to those with high levels of vulnerability and may be harmful to those who are resilient [32]. UK guidelines describe a three-tier approach to bereavement [33].

1. Most people manage without professional intervention, but may require information about the bereavement process.
2. Some people may require a formal mechanism to explore their experience. This can be done without involving professionals, for example, with self-help groups, volunteer befrienders and community groups.
3. Some people, including children and young people, will require specialist intervention. In different areas, this may come from psychology, mental health, or palliative care services.

Role of the Palliative Care Team

In many situations, the palliative care needs of patients with lung disease can be met by their respiratory teams. If teams are struggling to control a patient's symptoms, need help with psychological care, communication or difficult social situations, the palliative care team can provide help and support. This may be in the form of advice or direct assessment. A referral to palliative care services is based on need, not on diagnosis or prognosis.

Whether a patient is in hospital or at home, there will be a hospital, community, or integrated palliative care team available for advice or to assess a patient. This team has nurse specialists, consultants, and often social workers, physiotherapists, and occupation therapists. They have access to inpatient palliative care where more intensive palliative care or end of life care is required. Inpatient facilities come in the form of hospices or palliative care units within hospitals. Most can admit patients at any time of the day or night for emergencies. Day hospices play an important role for respiratory patients. In these settings, patients can attend a day service once a week with a group of other patients to receive symptom management, psychological care, specific interventions, rehabilitation, and peer support.

Final Thoughts

Managing the final stages of an illness requires active decision making and compassionate communication. Addressing physical, psychological, social, and spiritual issues greatly enhances a person's quality of life and this in turn impacts on the bereavement of their families. Most end of life care is delivered within families and communities, sometimes at home or in hospital. Specific palliative care services have an important role to play where the situation becomes more complex. End of life care is recognizing that it is less about dying and more about helping people to live as well as possible until they die. Rather than focusing on the end-point, it should focus on the path to get there. Sometimes by acknowledging and affirming patients' greatest fears and hopes, we can liberate individuals to cope and even flourish.

References

1. World Health Organization. http://www.who.int/cancer/palliative/definition/en/. Accessed Apr 2012.
2. Christakis N, Lamond E. Extent and determinants of error in doctors' prognoses in terminally ill patients: prospective cohort study. BMJ. 2000;320:469–72.
3. The Gold Standards Framework. 2011. www.goldstandardsframework.org.uk. Accessed Apr 2012.
4. Prognostic Indicator Guidance. 2011. www.goldstandardsframework.org.uk. Accessed Apr 2012.

5. Hill K, Muers M. Palliative care for patients with non-malignant end stage respiratory disease. Thorax. 2000;55:979–81.
6. Partridge M, Khatri A, Sutton L, et al. Palliative care for those with chronic lung disease. Chron Respir Dis. 2009;6:13–7.
7. Department of Health. End of Life Strategy – Promoting high quality care for all adults at the end of life. London: Department of Health; 2008.
8. Connors A, Dawson N, Thomas C. Outcomes following acute exacerbation of severe chronic obstructive lung disease. Am J Respir Crit Care Med. 1996;154:959–67.
9. Curtis J, Wenrich M, Carline J, et al. Patients' perspectives on physician skill in end of life care: differences between patients with COPD, cancer and AIDS. Chest. 2002;122:356–62.
10. Edmonds P, Karlsen S, Khan S, et al. A comparison of the palliative care needs of patients dying from chronic respiratory diseases and lung cancer. Palliat Med. 2001;15:287–95.
11. Curtis J, Engelberg R, Nielsen E, et al. Patient-physician communication about end of life care for patients with severe COPD. Eur Respir J. 2004;24:200–5.
12. Gore J, Brophy C, Greenstone M. How well do we care for patients with end stage chronic obstructive pulmonary disease (COPD)? A comparison of palliative care and quality of life in COPD and lung cancer. Thorax. 2000;55:1000–6.
13. British Medical Association. Decisions relating to cardiopulmonary resuscitation: a joint statement from the BMA, the Resuscitation Council, and the Royal College of Nursing. London: BMA; 2007.
14. National End of Life Care Programme. Capacity, care planning and advance care planning in life limiting illness – a guide for Health and Social Care Staff. London: Department of Health; 2011.
15. NHS End of Life Care Programme. Advance decisions to refuse treatment – a guide for Health and Social Care Staff. London: Department of Health; 2008.
16. Goodridge D. COPD as a life-limiting illness: advance care planning. Top Adv Pract Nurs. 2006;6:1–8.
17. e-ELCA. E-learning for Healthcare: e-End of Life Care for All. Department of Health; 2010. http://www.e-lfh.org.uk/projects/e-elca/index.html. Accessed Apr 2012.
18. NHS North East. Deciding right: an integrated approach to making care decisions in advance with children, young people and adults. NHS North East. 2011.
19. Obolensky L, Clark T, Matthew G, et al. A patient and relative centred evaluation of treatment escalation plans: a replacement for the do-not-resuscitate process. J Med Ethics. 2010;36:518–20.
20. Borgbjerg F, Nielsen K, Franks J. Experimental pain stimulates respiration and attenuates morphine-induced respiratory depression: a controlled study in human volunteers. Pain. 1996;64:123–8.
21. George R, Regnard C. Lethal opioids or dangerous prescribers? Palliat Med. 2007;21:77–80.
22. Skilbeck J, Mott L, Page H, et al. Palliative care in chronic obstructive airways disease: a needs assessment. Palliat Med. 1998;12:245–54.
23. European Association for Palliative Care. EAPC Taskforce on Spiritual Care in Palliative Care. 2010. www.eapcnet.eu. Accessed Apr 2012.
24. Morris M, Briant L, Chidgey-Clark J, et al. Bringing in care planning conversations for patients whose recovery is uncertain: learning from the AMBER care bundle. BMJ Support Palliat Care. 2011;1:72.
25. Wilkinson S, Ellershaw J. Care of the dying: a pathway to excellence. Oxford: Oxford University Press; 2003.
26. Marie Curie Palliative Care Institute. Liverpool care pathway for the dying patient. 2009. http://www.liv.ac.uk/mcpcil/liverpool-care-pathway/. Accessed Apr 2012.
27. Gomes B, Calanzani N, Higginson I. Local preferences and preferred place of death within England. Cicely Saunders International; 2011. www.cicelysaundersfoundation.org. Accessed Apr 2012.
28. National End of Life Care Programme/National End of Life Care Intelligence Network (NEoLCIN). Deaths from respiratory diseases: implications for end of life care in England. 2011. www.endoflifecare-intelligence.org.uk. Accessed Apr 2012.

29. Department for Work and Pensions. What to do after a death in England and Wales. London: Department for Work and Pensions; 2009.
30. Scottish Government. What to do after a death in Scotland. Edinburgh: The Scottish Government; 2008. www.scotland.gov.uk. Accessed Apr 2012.
31. Agnew A, Manktelow R, Taylor B, et al. Bereavement needs assessment in specialist palliative care: a review of the literature. Palliat Med. 2010;24:46–59.
32. Relf M, Machin L, Archer A. Guidance for bereavement needs assessment in palliative care. Help the Hospices. 2008. http://www.helpthehospices.org.uk. Accessed Apr 2012.
33. NICE. Guidance on Cancer Services: improving supportive and palliative care for adults with cancer. London: National Institute for Clinical Excellence; 2004.

Appendix

Respiratory Palliative Formulary

Abbreviations

CSCI   Continuous subcutaneous infusion by syringe driver over 24 h
IR   Immediate release (suspension, capsules or tablets)
LCP   Liverpool care pathway
MR   Modified release (tablets capsules or granules)

Pain

Opioid Analgesic Conversion Tables

In all opioid conversions, the convention is to describe the existing daily dose in terms of "24 hourly oral morphine equivalent" and then calculate the appropriate dose of the new drug from the conversions below (Tables A.1, A.2, and A.3).

Table A.1 Oral – oral or transdermal

	Potency ratio with morphine	Dose equivalence to 30 mg morphine
Codeine	1/10	300 mg codeine
Dihydrocodeine	1/10	300 mg dihydrocodeine
Tramadol	1/10	300 mg tramadol
Oxycodone	1.5	20 mg oxycodone
Hydromorphone	5	6 mg hydromorphone
Fentanyl (transdermal)	100	0.3 mg (i.e. 300 micrograms) fentanyl in 24 h (12 micrograms/h)

S.J. Bourke, E.T. Peel (eds.), *Integrated Palliative Care of Respiratory Disease*,
DOI 10.1007/978-1-4471-2230-2, © Springer-Verlag London 2013

Table A.2 Oral – subcutaneous

Oral	Divide by	Subcutaneous
Morphine (60 mg)	2	Morphine (30 mg)
Morphine (60 mg)	3	Diamorphine (20 mg)
Oxycodone (40 mg)	1.5	Oxycodone (30 mg)
Morphine (60 mg)	2	Oxycodone (30 mg)

Table A.3 Subcutaneous – subcutaneous

Subcutaneous	Divide by	Subcutaneous
Morphine (30 mg)	1	Oxycodone (30 mg)
Morphine (30 mg)	1.5	Diamorphine (20 mg)

Gabapentin Dosing

	Cautious	Usual
Day 1	100 mg at night	300 mg at night
Day 2	100 mg twice daily	300 mg twice daily
Day 3	100 mg three times daily	300 mg three times daily

Then titrate up at similar increments to maximum 900 mg three times daily, depending on symptoms and side effects.

Cough and Secretions

Cough Enhancement

Nebulized saline 0.9 % 5 ml four times daily
Nebulized DNAse 2,500 units (2.5 mg) once to twice daily (cystic fibrosis only)
Carbocisteine (capsules or suspension) 750 mg three times daily, orally

Central Cough Suppressants

Codeine linctus 15 mg (5 ml) four times daily (opioid naïve), orally
Morphine IR suspension 2.5–5 mg 4 hourly, orally
Methadone linctus 2 mg (5 ml) 12 hourly or
Equivalent pain rescue dose if already on strong opioid for pain

Peripheral Cough Suppressants

Simple linctus 5 ml four times daily

Removal of Secretions

Hyoscine hydrobromide 150–300 micrograms three times daily, orally
Hyoscine hydrobromide patch: 1 mg trans-dermal 72 hourly

Hemoptysis

Tranexamic Acid

1–1.5 g three times daily, orally or:
500 mg–1 g slow intravenous injection (over 5–10 min) three times daily, or:
25–50 mg/kg by intravenous infusion over 24 h

Breathlessness

Opioids

Opioid naïve:

Codeine phosphate 15 mg 6 hourly as required
Morphine IR susp 1–2.5 mg 4 hourly as required
Morphine MR tabs 10 mg once daily

On opioids already:

Usual IR rescue dose 4 hourly as required
End of life: Morphine sulphate 2.5 mg subcutaneously hourly as necessary.
Commence CSCI if two or more doses needed in 24 h

Benzodiazepines

1. Stable COPD: diazepam 2 mg once daily
2. Dyspnea associated with panic, requiring rapid palliation: lorazepam; 500 micrograms sublingually 6 hourly as required
3. End of life respiratory palliation: midazolam 5 mg/24 h CSCI titrated upwards as necessary

End of Life (LCP) Prescribing

For all of the end of life symptoms, as required dosing only is recommended, initially, if not already on the drug regularly. If two or more rescue doses are needed in 24 h, then commence CSCI as below.

Pain

If *already on opioids*: Convert 24 h oral morphine equivalent to appropriate dose given over 24 h by continuous subcutaneous infusion (CSCI). Rescue dose = 1/10–1/6 CSCI dose hourly as required

Escalate dose if two or more rescue doses in 24 h (by 1/3–1/2)

Opioid naïve: Start with morphine sulphate 2.5 mg or diamorphine 2.5 mg hourly as required. Commence CSCI: 10 mg/24 h if two or more rescue doses in 24 h.

Agitation

	CSCI (24 hourly)	Rescue
Haloperidol	1–3 mg (starting)	1.5 mg
Midazolam	5–10 mg (starting)	2.5–5 mg
Levomepromazine	50 mg	12.5–25 mg

Nausea and Vomiting

If already on an antiemetic, then convert to CSCI at the same total oral dose. Otherwise:
Cyclizine 50 mg subcutaneously 6 hourly as necessary, max 150 mg in 24 h, or:
Haloperidol 1.5 mg subcutaneously 6 hourly as necessary, max three doses, or:
Levomepromazine 6.25 mg subcutaneously 6 hourly as necessary.

Death Rattle

	CSCI (24 hourly)	Rescue
Hyoscine hydrobromide	1.2–2.4 mg	400 micrograms
Hyoscine butylbromide	60–120 mg	20 mg
Glycopyrronium	600 micrograms–1.2 mg	200 micrograms

Licensed Drugs Prescribed in an Unlicensed (Off-label) Way in Palliative Care

Drug	Off-label use
Afentanil	Subcutaneous
Amitriptyline	Neuropathic pain
	Bladder spasm
Baclofen	Hiccup
Carbamazepine	Neuropathic pain
Clonazepam	Neuropathic pain
	Restless legs syndrome
	Terminal restlessness
Dexamethasone	Appetite stimulant
	Bowel obstruction
	Dyspnea
	Nausea and vomiting
	Bone and nerve compression pain
	Spinal cord compression

Drug	Off-label use
Diamorphine	Painful skin lesions – topical
	Dyspnea
Erythromycin	Prokinetic agent
Etamsylate	Prophylaxis and control of hemorrhages from small blood vessels
Fentanyl	Subcutaneous
Fluoxetine	Anxiety
Gabapentin	Malignant bone pain
	Restless legs syndrome
Gtn spray	Smooth muscle spasm pain
Glycopyrronium	Hypersalivation
	Nausea and vomiting associated with bowel obstruction
	Smooth muscle spasm
	Sweating associated with cancer
	Terminal secretions
	Unlicensed subcutaneously
Granisetron	Nausea and vomiting – drug induced and cancer related, refractory
	Unlicensed subcutaneously
Haloperidol	Delirium
	Nausea and vomiting
	Unlicensed subcutaneously
Hyoscine butylbromide	Nausea and vomiting associated with bowel obstruction
	Smooth muscle spasm – colic
	Sweating
	Terminal secretions
	Unlicensed subcutaneously
Hyoscine hydrobromide	Hypersalivation
	Smooth muscle spasm – colic
	Sweating
	Terminal secretions
Ketamine	Refractory chronic pain
	Unlicensed subcutaneously
	Unlicensed orally
	Incident pain
Ketorolac	Short-term management of cancer pain
	Unlicensed subcutaneously
Levomepromazine	Unlicensed indications
	Psychosis (by injection)
	Nausea and vomiting (tablets)
Lidocaine patch	Post-thoracotomy pain
	Post-mastectomy pain
	Localized neuropathic and muscular pain
Loperamide	Bowel colic
	Reduction of stoma output (topically on mouth ulcers)
Lorazepam	Dyspnea
	Unlicensed sublingually
Medroxyprogesterone	Anorexia and cachexia

Drug	Off-label use
Methylphenidate	Cancer-related fatigue
	Depression
Midazolam	Dyspnea
	Epilepsy
	Hiccup
	Major hemorrhage
	Myoclonus
	Status epilepticus
	Terminal agitation or anxiety
	Unlicensed subcutaneously
Mirtazapine	Appetite
	Nausea and vomiting
	Pruritus
Morphine	Painful skin lesions – topical
	Mucositis – topical
	Cough
	Dyspnea
Nifedipine	Smooth muscle spasm pain
	Intractable hiccup
Olanzapine	Nausea and vomiting
	Delirium
	Terminal agitation (refractory to conventional treatment)
Ondansetron	Nausea and vomiting
	Pruritus(opioid induced, cholestatic, uremic)
	Unlicensed subcutaneously
Oxycodone	Dyspnea
Phenobarbital	Terminal agitation (in patients not controlled conventionally)
	Unlicensed subcutaneously
Pregabalin	Malignant bone pain, sleep improvement
Risperidone	Delirium, anti-emetic (refractory nausea and vomiting)
	Major depression
Sodium valproate	Unlicensed subcutaneously
Sucralfate	Surface bleeding
Tranexamic acid	Prophylaxis and control of hemorrhage from small blood vessels
	Bleeding from wounds (topical)
Zoledronic acid	Bone pain

Unlicensed Drugs in Palliative Care

Cyclizine	Unlicensed – suppositories available
Gabapentin	Unlicensed liquid available
Glycopyrronium	Unlicensed tablets available
Hydromorphone	Unlicensed – injection
Ketorolac	Unlicensed liquid available
Levomepromazine	6 mg tablet – unlicensed
Midazolam	Epistat – unlicensed buccal liquid

Index